'Lois Oppenheim offers a brilliant consideration of what makes us human by investigating the question of why we value art. Her interdisciplinary approach through aesthetics, neuroscience, and psychoanalysis models the value of integrative thinking on an understanding of how we approach the crisis of not knowing what we need to know, the crisis of uncertainty. Her focus on the grounding of consciousness in feeling argues strongly against a reductive deterministic approach to human experience. Her presentation of the interrelation of curiosity, creativity, and crisis inspires hope for the future of humankind in the context of sociopolitical crisis.'

Harriet Wolfe, M.D., Past President, International Psychoanalytical Association

'At last, a neuroscience of aesthetics based on a systematic exploration of the basic emotions.'

Oliver Turnbull, Prof of Neuropsychology, Bangor University Wales, UK

'Deftly combining neuroscience, psychoanalysis and art, Lois Oppenheim opens up new ways of thinking about creativity. Challenging deterministic understandings of the aesthetically-engaged mind—whether in artists and writers or viewers and readers—she brings her immense erudition to bear on questions of what impels "the curiosity and creativity that characterize human experience." Taking the mind to be an active agent, and imagination a human need, Oppenheim writes clearly, thoughtfully and with urgent concern about the crises jeopardizing the artistic freedoms she champions.'

Nancy Princenthal, author, *Agnes Martin: Her Life and Art and Unspeakable Acts: Women, Art, and Sexual Violence in the 1970s.*

Neuroaesthetics and Psychoanalysis

This book looks at the fundamental question of why we take pleasure in art through a relatively new perspective of neuroaesthetics and explores the close links between cognitive and affective processes used in understanding art and science.

Drawing on the new and rapidly developing school of neuroaesthetics, the author explores the meaning of mind in the context of both creation and viewing. She considers the meaning of the affective experience of color and form, as well as the meaning of "modern" and its aftermath, all within the context of pleasure and its source. This book further enframes the pleasure of aesthetic experience in the embodiment of mind defined by the concept of drive. It is an exploration of how the mind becomes what it is, of its comprehensive relation to the neuroperceptual, to feeling, to ambiguity and uncertainty that allows for an understanding of what would more tellingly be termed 'neuropsychoaesthetics'.

With insights drawn from the latest neuroscientific findings and a deep understanding of both artistic and scientific thinking, this is key reading for psychoanalysts, psychotherapists, and anyone wanting to understand the human mind better.

Lois Oppenheim is Professor Emerita at Montclair State University, where she was named University Distinguished Scholar. She is also on the faculty of the New York Psychoanalytic Society and Institute. She has previously authored or edited fifteen books, including *Imagination from Fantasy to Delusion* which was awarded the Courage to Dream Prize from the American Psychoanalytic Association.

The Routledge Neuropsychoanalysis Series

Series editor: Mark Solms

The attempt to integrate the findings and methods of psychoanalysis with those of the neurological sciences can be said to have begun in 1895, with Freud's Project for a Scientific Psychology. Ongoing, sporadic efforts continued throughout the 20th century. However, the field really took off when the journal Neuropsychoanalysis was founded in 1999 and the International Neuropsychoanalysis Society was established in 2000. Ever since, a themed annual congress has been held in different cities around the world. Today, it is fair to say that these efforts have generated the most rapidly growing and influential body of knowledge and clinical practice in the broader field of psychoanalysis.

The establishment of this book series in 2023 marked another important milestone in the development of the field. Under the editorship of Mark Solms, the co-chair of the International Neuropsychoanalysis Society, it publishes books by leading proponents - and critics - of neuropsychoanalysis. The books in this series focus not only on the scientific findings of neuropsychoanalysis and on its theoretical yield, but also on its history, its philosophical implications and its clinical practice, as well as its ramifications for neighbouring disciplines and for the mental and neurological sciences as a whole.

The Unconscious in Neuroscience and Psychoanalysis: On Lacan and Freud
Marco Máximo Balzarini

Explorations Between Psychoanalysis and Neuroscience: At the Edge of Mind and Brain
David D. Olds

Neuroscience and the Death Drive: The Nature of Symptoms, from Formulation to Treatment
Adrian Perkel

Neuroaesthetics and Psychoanalysis: Curiosity, Creativity, and Crisis
Lois Oppenheim

Neuroaesthetics and Psychoanalysis

Curiosity, Creativity, and Crisis

Lois Oppenheim

Routledge
Taylor & Francis Group
LONDON AND NEW YORK

Designed cover image: John Opper, Untitled (AM6–18), 1976, acrylic on canvas, 34 x 38 inches. © Jane Opper and Joseph Opper

First published 2026
by Routledge
4 Park Square, Milton Park, Abingdon, Oxon OX14 4RN

and by Routledge
605 Third Avenue, New York, NY 10158

Routledge is an imprint of the Taylor & Francis Group, an informa business

British Library Cataloguing-in-Publication Data
A catalogue record for this book is available from the British Library

ISBN: 978-1-032-93622-2 (hbk)
ISBN: 978-1-032-93358-0 (pbk)
ISBN: 978-1-003-56675-5 (ebk)

DOI: 10.4324/9781003566755

Typeset in Times New Roman
by Taylor & Francis Books

For Sarah and Keith

Contents

Figures

Preface

Mark Rothko's "search for unity, and the society's as well, may be an attempt to fend off an incipient existential crisis – to find consistency and meaning in the face of increasing entropy."[1]

As I neared completion of this book, I came across this statement by the American abstract painter's son. One cannot but be struck by its correspondence with the Free Energy Principle that originated in physics and has been adopted by many in neuroscience to explain the minimization of uncertainty, the modeling of our experience of the world for prediction and thereby learning, the unifying process that allows for the avoidance of such crisis. The formulations of those, like Karl Friston, who focus on the perceptual and cognitive gains and losses of what is termed Predictive Processing were, I was informed by Christopher Rothko, unknown to him. One could hardly hope for a more fortuitous validation of a book's explorative purpose: the uncovering of where it is that art and science meet.

L.O.
New York, 2025

Note

1 C. Rothko, "Introduction," in M. Rothko, *The Artist's Reality* (New Haven & London, 2004), xxi.

Acknowledgments

Many are those to be thanked for innumerable reasons: Christa Balzert, Geneviève Chevallier, Michael Coffey, the late Sidney Feshbach, Christopher Rothko, Rebecca Smith, and Silvia Baron Supervielle, among others. Once again, I am immensely grateful to my husband, Ellis Oppenheim, for his exceeding patience and equanimity.

Introduction

The phenomenologist Jacques Garelli wrote in 2005 of the use of theories borrowed by philosophy from thermodynamics and quantum physics. These concerned "the contemporary conception of beings" and the concept of the pre-individual to which it relates. In so doing, he reflected "on the exemplary prudence of Niels Bohr and Werner Heisenberg" each time they confronted the problem of "the philosophical status (but which could also be called the 'mode of being') of the quantum particle." This fundamentally ontological concern was "central," Garelli noted, "to the meditations of these physicists" and he deemed it important to recall a "pressing question" posed by Heisenberg to Bohr involving a problem relevant not only to physics and not simply "as soon as the question of beings is posed, but also as soon as the philosopher – acknowledging that the dominant state of nature is not matter but energy – calls into question the capacity of our mind to 'understand' the components of this phenomenon." The question was as follows: "If the inner structure of the atom is as closed to descriptive accounts as you say, if we really lack a language for dealing with it, how can we ever hope to understand atoms?" As reported by Heisenberg, Bohr hesitated briefly before replying, "I think we may yet be able to do so. But in the process we may have to learn what the word 'understanding' really means."[1]

*

Where Art Meets Science was initially the subtitle of this book. A primary objective in the early stages of its writing was to identify a juncture in need of recognition. My intention was to demonstrate *how* an insufficiently acknowledged association is illustrative of our era and *why* it is critical to our understanding of the destabilization with which, in so many arenas, we currently contend. It was inspired, in part, by the devaluation of the intellectual in the 21st century (and the concomitant quasi-disappearance of the humanities from higher education; indeed, the reduced valorization of higher education altogether) that constitutes a crisis of curiosity and creative thinking due, to some extent, to the convergence in question. And it was inspired, in part, by an increasing awareness of what Bruno Latour described as follows: "the sciences

DOI: 10.4324/9781003566755-1

are now and will remain from now on so intermingled with the entire culture that we need to turn to the humanities to understand how they really function."[2] This was certainly not to imply that science is any less a product of curiosity or creative reflection than what is more commonly associated with imagination (i.e., aesthetic experience), but that the linear causality defining its parameters was increasingly an impediment to the kind of "enlightenment" remediation, the rational thinking (or, to put it more colloquially, a coming to our senses!) so lacking in this period of the incomprehensibly austere and progressively (or seemingly so) inhumane. What ultimately ensued was a question of just *what* this art-science confluence is, a significantly increased appreciation of the depth of the intersection itself, and a need to "understand" how "understanding" might impact the crisis of uncertainty with which we now contend.

The interrelation of art and science was already intriguing to me some years ago as I began to dig into what I termed (and ultimately titled a book[3]) "a curious intimacy," the relation between art and neuropsychoanalysis. My interest lay in the complex implications of the newly founded discipline of neuropsychoanalysis for our understanding of the making and appreciation of literature, painting, and dance (with the art of Samuel Beckett, Paul Klee, and Martha Graham the exemplars whose work I explored). More recently, however, what has become abundantly clear is that the distinction between affective and cognitive neuroscience, at the crux of the neuropsychoanalytically framed investigation of the aesthetic, overshadows the primacy of their interrelation in the pleasure we take in literary and visual art. Or, to put it more precisely, the distinction between cognition and affect, with the neuroscientific perspectives deriving from each, simplistically eclipses the *source* of the one as residing in the other. And it is the identification of this interconnection – the detection of the one as dependent upon the other, *it is detection of the affective as the very foundation of the cognitive* – that allows for the neuropsychoanalytic appreciation of aesthetic experience.

For much of the 1990s and early 2000s, neuroaesthetics was grounded in how beauty intersects with the workings of the visual brain. Semir Zeki brought recognition to the neural anatomy, the visual circuitry, governing both the execution and reception of painting and sculpture. Vittorio Gallese brought recognition to the neural mechanism of mirroring, the systemic activation of neural networks in response to artistic expression. Subliminal recognition on the part of the viewer and thereby communication with the viewed led Gallese to the notion of "embodied simulation," the notion of an empathetically framed, motoric resonance at play in the experiencing of art. It was Antonio Damasio, Jaak Panksepp, and Mark Solms, however, who brought attention to the workings of those neural processes as essential to affect, consciousness, and the relation between them. It was Damasio, Panksepp, and Solms whose interest in feeling, if not in aesthetic creation or reception as such, revealed the role of emotion in cognition, the part played by affect in awareness, paving the way for others more focused on aesthetic experience to appreciate what Solms calls "the *functional organization* of the brain as a whole"[4] and thus the subjective and dynamic dimensions implicated in the making and valuing of art.[5]

There are those today who, like Lisa Feldman Barrett, in privileging cognition over emotion, in ignoring the dependence of the one upon the other, share the view that imagination is dependent upon what is known, those who share, in other words, a *deterministic* perspective on creativity. Exemplified by what Barrett calls "the Picasso Principle," the idea that Picasso could only create cubism by having knowledge of classical painting, imagination is relegated to the realm of the cerebral and thus aesthetic experience is for them not as much about the subjectivity of feeling, whatever the source of that feeling, as about what one knows. "Creativity is a skill," Barrett has said, a skill "that is learnable."[6] If this is so, what is the *meaning of pleasure* in the context of aesthetics? Where does neuronal activity, the subjective arousal experienced by artist and viewer alike, come into the (metaphorical) picture?

As the mind alone is the possessor of subjectivity, the vehicle of consciousness, it stands to reason that it is the mental function of the brain that is the system by which feeling is felt. This is to say that *feeling* defines the mind-brain relation, that it is their unifying feature. Indeed, this is what Solms has dedicated much of his recent written work to demonstrating. Just what, however, is the mind? How is it to be defined? Hardly an unexplored topic, of course, but more to the point: How does it *become* what it is? This is the question with which to begin a book such as this if one takes issue, as I do, with the *determinist* perspective of the cognitivist who claims knowledge precedes creativity, knowing precedes imagining, as opposed to the idea that it is curiosity, the actual search for knowledge, that impels the imagination. How might we understand the dynamic functioning of the mentalization involved in the creative process? How might we understand the energic mentalizing activity from which creativity (whether in science or art) flows? These are questions that will inform what follows Chapter One, a chapter whose focus on the "becoming" of mind is meant to set the stage for an exploration of aesthetic experience, of what it is constituted and how it might be psychodynamically comprehended. Whether in science or art, the relation between curiosity and creativity is complex but certain. And both, in a sense, are driven by a form of crisis: the very fact of *not* knowing, its psychological, neurochemical, and neurobiological consequences; the implicit need for knowledge upon which our very existence depends.

In a recent paper entitled "Computational Psychiatry: From Synapses to Sentience," the British neuroscientist Karl Friston marvels "at how a common, computational, narrative can bring molecular biologists and clinical neuroscientists to the same table." The narrative to which he refers is that of the brain as an organ of extrapolation and anticipation, a narrative in which "neuronal activity encodes expectations about the causes of sensory input" and continually updates them to minimize errors of prediction.[7] To that table, however wondrous already, I would additionally bring neuroaestheticians and neuropsychoanalysts, for predictive coding, as this computational narrative is known, has now made its way into aesthetics and psychoanalysis contributing much to our understanding of each while also raising questions about certain conclusions, conclusions erroneously inferred by some, or so it would seem.

Neuroaesthetics and neuropsychoanalysis are two relatively young disciplines linked more by the subjectivity of affect, the actuality of emotion and its psychoanalytic implications, than their shared anatomically related prefix might have us believe. Aesthetic experience, like the psychoanalytic understanding of mind, is a domain in which the dynamic constituents of pleasure and unpleasure implicate the psychic and the corporeal alike. That neuroaesthetics integrates what is theoretically and pragmatically known of the mind with what is theoretically and pragmatically known of the brain – much as psychoanalysis, beginning with Freud (a neurologist and neuroscientist, lest one forget), views the mind and body as dynamically interconnected – serves as a means of understanding aesthetic experience. Technically speaking, *neuroaesthetics* connotes the experiencing of art by the nervous system while *psychoaesthetics* relates to the psychodynamic experience of making and responding to art. Conjoined, however, they comprise what might be called *neuropsychoaesthetics*, a term (to my knowledge, not in use as of yet but one that, however cumbersome, now should be) designating what psychoanalysis brings to the neuroaesthetic front. Focusing primarily on painting as exemplary of the aesthetic domain, this book is an exploration of the ontology of aesthetic experience. Visual and literary art, music, theater, dance: Each is a function of feeling such that three terms fundamental to that ontology come to the fore.

*

Crisis. A word emblematic of our time. Or, rather, crises, for indeed there are many: Humanitarian crises, ecological crises, public health crises, economic crises, and more. Or "krisis" as it appears in Edmund Husserl's 1936 unfinished work targeting the critical state of the European sciences, the word itself imagistically projecting something harsher with the k of the German and of its Greek origin. In his final work, *The Crisis of European Sciences and Transcendental Phenomenology*, the philosopher urgently appeals to his reader to attend to what has been termed the "scientific, moral and existential" crises of his time: The crisis "brought on by the positivity of the sciences," the "crisis in the human sciences" for being modeled on the exact sciences, the "crisis in contemporary culture ('a radical life-crisis of European humanity')," among others, as described by Dermot Moran. Together they constituted for Husserl one larger crisis: "the failure of European rationality, despite the enormous advances of the sciences in the technological domination of the world and in the technical organization of society, to have supplied a cure for social and psychic illness of the time."[8]

Some twelve years after Husserl's *The Crisis*, another of the most important works of the twentieth century was published: Jean-Paul Sartre's *What is Literature?*. Composed of three independent essays, it poses in each a question that could hardly be more fundamental: "What is writing?" "Why write?" and "For whom does one write?" One scarcely need wonder why Sartre explored these questions when he did. Following on the heels of the Second World War, he was impelled to probe the existential themes of responsibility and commitment (themes previously studied by him in *Nausea, Being and Nothingness*, and elsewhere) in the implicit context of an ideal free society. "To speak is to act," Sartre exclaimed; "anything which one names is already no longer quite the same; it has lost its innocence."[9]

Soon to become identified as the hallmark of Sartre's writing was the employment of literature for, as François Noudelmann has put it, "the benefit of politics."[10] Yet, as Noudelmann so rightly notes, Sartre's notion of commitment was nothing of the sort. A great many of his writings stress the irreducibility of the literary and visual arts and today we would do well to rethink Sartre as antidotal to what Noudelmann describes as the "*determinisms* that are returning in force."[11] If Sartre's thinking in this masterful work appeared for a time outmoded, as having lost its relevance, today it reveals a significance that could not be more germane to the crises of our time, a significance that not only should not but must not be overlooked. Like the most astute intellectuals of the mid-to-late twentieth century, Sartre both reflected and inspired reflection, was aware and sought to render others aware. He prized the capacity and the adventuresomeness of the mind and, like those who expressed it in works of literary and visual art, despaired of the deterministic banality in which it could become stuck. So, too, the absurdist playwrights in France and the pop artists in the U.S. who displayed mid-century the "crisis of thought [...] manifested by a crisis of language,"[12] as Eugene Ionesco put it, convention having come to dominate life where determinism reigns.

Just what is this determinism and what are its effects? Noudelmann notes two of particular significance: the determinism of economic thinking "which would have us accept that economic liberalization is the only future for the planet" and scientific determinism meant to persuade us "that the workings of thought can be reduced to the workings of the neurones." Sartre, he tells us, "always fought against this kind of reductionism."[13] Others, Simone Weil and Hannah Arendt, to cite but two, fought hard against any reductionist ideology ensuing from the deterministic limiting of active citizenship. Simone de Beauvoir and feminist thinkers long inspired by her struggled against the reductionism of gender determinism. Susan Sontag fought any reductionist ideology that limited our understanding of aesthetics and the phenomenology of art by way of a determinist view of meaning in the novel, in plays, and in film as opposed to consideration of *how* they are what they are. Most recently, some in neuroscience are seeking to define how the mechanism of plasticity, the operational alterations (both structural and functional) resulting from experience, deconstruct the determinism of genetics and epigenetics. What psychoanalyst François Ansermet along with neuroscientist Pierre Magistretti have offered, for instance, is the framing as plastic – which is to say "neither determined nor undetermined" insofar as plasticity is a reworking, synchronic and diachronic, of neural circuits – of what they term the process of becoming.[14] Psychoanalytically, neuroscientifically, and philosophically speaking, becoming is what connects the evolving with the intermittent, the continuous with the discontinuous, to account for the experiential. In defiance of a deterministic understanding, it will be my purpose to show that experience of the aesthetic is not reducible to neural activity however engaged it is by the making or reception of art.

Other determinisms come to mind, but it is perhaps what has been called by Alice Jardine "an allergy to thinking" that best defines the determinist mentality confronting us today. And it is Julia Kristeva who perhaps battles most fiercely this "incapacity to think – especially when thinking is uncomfortable, challenging, or even dangerous" and the "resistance to re-thinking, to remembering – the loss of historical memory [that] leads to the banality of evil,"[15] as famously described by Arendt in her 1963 study of Adolph Eichmann. The effect of such a determinism has been a deleterious alteration of "the figure of the intellectual," as Noudelmann puts it: "Instead of being a moral or political conscience intellectuals have become 'experts' who make assessments and stand in the shadow of the authorities."[16] Indeed, we bear witness today to an anti-intellectualism, such as intellectualism once was, to an anti-humanitarianism even, and to a reinforcement of the determinism that reduces both integrity and imagination while constituting a crisis of unfathomable scope.

Yet, there is also this: "The crisis of understanding in the physical sciences and its consequences in the philosophical conception of beings,"[17] to cite once again Garelli. Writing of "the reevaluation of Niels Bohr's principle of complementarity," the "original interpretation of Heisenberg's uncertainty principle," and "a reevaluation of the interpretation of the introduction of statistical calculus into the mathematical formulation of this principle" as offered by the philosopher Gilbert Simondon, Garelli acknowledges Simondon's understanding of transduction as "the effort of thinking, in one and the same unity, 'the object' of research and the movement of knowledge that drives it."[18] In recognition of this concept as fundamental both to science and art, of the need to obfuscate the Aristotelian duality of matter and form in favor of the emergence that unites them, Simondon stresses the need to "seek to know the individual through individuation rather than individuation through the individual."[19] His thinking constitutes what Garelli terms "the crisis of meaning that has shaken the scientific and philosophical problematic." A "procedure of the mind as it discovers," transduction "consists in following *being in its genesis*, in carrying out the genesis of thought at the same time as the genesis of the object is carried out."[20] This is a crisis owing to the insufficient grasp on the part of science – and, as we shall see in the chapters that follow, on a segment of neuroscience as well – of the processes of individuation, the notion of the pre-individual these processes entail and the becoming of mind and maturation as inseparable from, but irreducible to, the physiology of the brain. This is a "crisis of meaning" that necessitates a reconsideration of aesthetic experience outside the dichotomization of artwork and viewer, reader, or listener and a re-situating of such experience in the frame of what comes into being.

And then there is this – The crisis more fundamentally existential than any other, the one with which we interact at every moment and in every modality from perception to action: homeostasis. More accurately described as a potential crisis than an actual crisis, the crisis of homeostatic stability is one we face continually by virtue of our constitution as human beings, by virtue of our cerebral anatomy, its neuronal connectivity and processing. Principles such as predictive coding, active inference, and the minimization of free energy – all paradigms of perception, learning, and behavior – are increasingly replacing our conception of the brain as a passive organ in favor of one actively generating images and hypotheses against which sensory evidence is continually put to the test.[21] As such, they are principles which account for the curiosity and creativity that characterize human experience. Is the advent of neuroscience's increasing acceptance, as the tools with which its various hypotheses may be evaluated become ever more available, contributing to an anti-humanistic determinism? Or is an interdisciplinarity – a nearing of the objectives of cognitive and affective neuroscience, say, or of neuroscience and psychoanalysis, or neuroscience and aesthetics – able to thwart off the risk of such a determinism by its integration of the *how* with the *why*?

Creativity. Creative process – as a means of revealing the uniquely subjective experience of every individual, the potentiality and agency of the self, and its capacity for intersubjective engagement – is devalued as unspeakable atrocities deflate the very value of being human, of the humanitarian and, consequentially, the humanities as well. Creative process – as a means of unveiling, a means of revealing, through the co-construction of the aesthetic object by writer and reader or painter and viewer the freedom inherent within all – is particularly pertinent at this time. Humanitarian crises of unfathomable proportions in Israel/Palestine, Syria, Afghanistan, Ukraine, the Congo, and elsewhere in the world; crises of violence such as arose in Washington, D.C. on January 6, 2021 and increasingly result from anti-Semitic, anti-Islamic, anti-Asian, and white supremacist acts, from deep racially prejudicial divides; climate change and other ecological crises; public health and personal crises before devastating loss and fear – all impel us to question the relation of crisis to thinking, to creative thinking, to creative output in science, in the arts, in whatever the domain. But not without implicating at once several other questions: What really is the meaning of creativity and whence does it emerge? What do we mean by creative thinking: thinking that is original or something more? How are verbal and visual artmaking impacted by a world in crisis, by an individual in crisis? Are many inspired to create in the effort to make a difference, as did Sartre? Or does despair before the feeling of helplessness impede such activist productivity? Or cause the curious to lose whatever it is that in better times stimulates their inquisitiveness, their questioning, by way of the verbal or visual image? Or even cause one to cede to the shame of finding oneself in a position to be creative while others, in almost incomprehensible numbers, are ill and dying?

For some, the world in crisis is no longer familiar, but uncanny, *unheimlich* as Freud observed, an effect that – in going well beyond the familiar while re-finding it within the guise of the unfamiliar – results from an effacing of "the distinction between imagination and reality."[22] "Surreal" is how many think of it. For some, there is solace to be found in making art under the weight of crisis. Yet, if art at this critical moment in the history of our civilization, at this moment when multiple crises are convergent, provides protection, embodying, as it does, what Kristeva terms "universal singularities" – "a universalism," as Jardine has explained, "based on the recognition of the irreducible singularity of each and every one of us"[23] – it also reveals a vulnerability, a defenselessness before a politico-social reality, to cite but one example, that requires a return to the very notion of freedom of which Sartre sought to make us aware. It requires a return to what Sartre in the 1940s and Kristeva today proclaim is *the very value of imagination*, however simplistic that moral imperative may appear.

Freud's theory of sublimation, as is well known, situated the value of imagination in the redirecting of unacceptable urges toward the socially acceptable. But is one to take from this that a degree of perversion, or even simply conflict, is necessarily the primary ingredient in or the motivational force behind the creative process? Is one to take from Freud's thinking on sublimation that art is reducible to adaptation, to the redirecting of impulse, to therapeutic remediation? Many are those who have explored from one or another psychoanalytic perspective the corrective value of artistic creation, the rectification of aspects of early development and interpersonal relationships. I will discuss the relation of the artist to the artwork throughout this book, but it is neither the notion of unconscious conflict nor that of interpersonal phenomena that motivates its writing. Rather, what I wish to explore is another kind of what has been termed the "constructive aspect of the artistic process." Writing of the work of psychoanalyst Phyllis Greenacre from more than a half century ago, work which remains relevant to our thinking on art yet today, Volney P. Gay noted that "the work of art is an organized and organizing achievement in which creative persons find within sensual experience moments in which the world and the self cohere."[24] A fundamentally interdisciplinary exploration appears required to achieve any real understanding of in what that coherence consists.

Both Sartre and Kristeva found in writing – and also in psychoanalysis (with one engaging in critical writing from an existential psychoanalytic viewpoint, the other practicing clinically as well as writing) – the means to exercise the right of every human being to what Jardine terms "a living psychic space" and validation of the belief that "psychic death is about the death of the imaginary – a death from which only a culture of revolt can save us."[25] Might this, in some sense, be seen an expression of revolt against the uncanniness of the current state in which we find ourselves, against the lack of familiarity, the unhomeliness, associated not only with the manifest crises referred to above, but with the latent crisis that is the reductionist mode of thinking, the *determinism*, characteristic of much of the world, certainly of the Western world, of the twenty-first century? Is the revolt not essentially aimed at a *deterministic* mode of thinking characterized, above all else, by a materialistic, quasi-algorithmic redefining of what it is to be human?[26] Are the crises with which we are faced today limited to war, to ecology, to the racial and other forms of marginalization of long standing (in the now ironically named United States, but elsewhere as well)? Is there not, in fact, another, perhaps more primary, crisis underlying the rise of extreme conservativism, of the authoritarianism that silences difference and dialogue in one fell swoop, and the other crises as well? Are we really prey to clearly distinct crises – those of political oppression that has extended well into the ravages of war, of an uncanniness before a global pandemic whose exigencies erupted in stunning surges of violence – or is there an underlying feature, an as yet unnamed reductionistic determinism that is simultaneously cause and effect of an amalgamated, while not existentially cohesive, state of being?

Interestingly, Husserl attributed the crises of which he wrote to, as Moran explains, "the crucial neglect of *the subjective contribution to the experience of the world*" (emphasis mine). He located the solution to the crises he identified as interrelated in "transcendental phenomenology with its secure and grounded clarification of the concept of *subjectivity*."[27] "Un cri de douleur est signe de la douleur qui le provoque," Sartre declared in the first of his three essays referred to above, "Mais un chant de douleur est à la fois la douleur elle-même et autre chose que la douleur" ("A cry of pain is the sign of the grief which provokes it. But a song of pain is both pain itself and something other than pain").[28] Distinguishing between the language of poetry and that of prose, he defined the poet as one who refuses to utilize language, opting instead to unveil both the subjectivity of their own creative experience and that of the reader in an intersubjective mode of engagement intrinsic to all art whatever the form.[29] Like Husserl, Sartre sought in subjectivity the therapeutic solution to the illness of inhumanity, the malevolence of the human being confronting their own kind. Like Husserl and others he influenced – Martin Heidegger and Maurice Merleau-Ponty most important among them – he saw the experience of the subject, the focus of his existential phenomenology, in terms of the immediacy of its contact with the world. We are not in the world, but of it, as Garelli (following Merleau-Ponty) reminded us, the world not being an object of knowledge, but the field of greatest intimacy whereby we constitute our self.[30] Kristeva as well locates the potential for the kind of revolt needed to counter the crises that plague us precisely within the subjectivity of the written word, within the opportunities afforded by literature and the other arts to counter the "psychic death [that] is about the death of the imaginary,"[31] as Jardine puts it. The arts, like psychoanalysis, combat "the suffocation of psychic space"[32] that results in multiple forms of the surreal, the uncanny, the violence and barbarism with which we are currently contending.

One can only wonder, be curious, about how attention to subjectivity, to the existential freedom that lies therein – subjectivity as discussed by Husserl, Sartre, Kristeva, and others, as demonstrated by literary and visual artists alike – might take us *beyond the pervasive if destabilizing determinism to the respect for human experience.* One can only wonder, be curious, about what it is we do when we modify our sensibilities, when we create literary and visual art. One can only wonder, be curious, about the relation between the within and the without, the relation between the subjective and objective viewpoints that are driven not by this or by that determinative system, but an integrative discourse fueled by creative thinking about and inquisitive exploration of the intersections at hand. Indeed, what is the relation between creativity and curiosity? Just what is curiosity itself?

Curiosity. With racial tensions, anti-Semitism, and other exclusionary distortions of our universality – with their accompanying violence proliferating with the voracious spread of populism, of unspeakable killings of schoolchildren and the torture of hostages, proliferating like the virus that spread throughout the world at breakneck speed – we think about the relation of a destabilized (profoundly uncivilized) civilization and currents in literature and painting, the reasons for making art, why art has always been with us (regardless of culture) and what art is. Clearly, the notion of freedom is to be reconsidered in light of the present situation. Clearly, the notions of commitment and responsibility are to be reconsidered in light of the inhumanity at hand. Sartre's voice, the voice of the voiceless – "the voice of Jews, Black Americans, Koreans, Congolese, Algerians, Vietnamese, Palestinians" as Noudelmann put it[33] – is not to be relegated to the past. And it is within the very voice proclaiming now as before the need to resist, the need to recognize a foundational freedom and its moral concomitance, the need to revive humanitarianism, humanism, and the humanities that the valorization of imagination itself is to be found: "Parler c'est agir" ("To speak is to act"), wrote Sartre in 1948.[34] And, two years prior, "vous êtes libre, choisissez, c'est-à-dire inventez" ("you are free, choose, that is to say invent").[35]

Imagining, in itself, is an expression of curiosity, a response to uncertainty, a questioning *why?*. Whatever the domain, it requires releasing the hold on determinism (be it economic, scientific, technocratic, or other) and the dichotomizing – brain/mind, physiology/psychology, nature/nurture, liberal/conservative, and so on – determinism implies. Acknowledgement of this allows for integrative dialogue, interdisciplinary and imaginative discourse wherein humanism resides. In a word, the destruction of freedom as agency, freedom as desire, and freedom as authentic social interaction constitutes a potential for psychic calamity, for the ruination of curiosity and thereby creativity and the intersubjectivity creativity implies.

In what follows I will consider the "crisis of meaning" (as Garelli called it), the crisis that has shaken the physical sciences and had significant consequences in the philosophical understanding of the conception of being.[36] I will consider what constituted for Husserl the "scientific, moral and existential" crises of his time which involves *turning from the determinism of positivism toward the subjectivity that is experience.* This will entail looking, first, as I said above, at the emergence of mind and, specifically, at the becoming of mind as put forth in an unpublished (as decided by the authors themselves) but highly significant study that predates, but impressively anticipates, more recent developments in neuroaesthetics and neuropsychoanalysis. As the mind-body problem continues to struggle against the notion of an inherent duality (as opposed to a monist position favoring two views of a single phenomenon[37]), the discourse of human development similarly struggles against the nature vs. nurture bifurcation that has long dominated any determination of how the mind of an individual becomes just what it is. Yet, as we shall see by way of the study, some of whose findings are to be examined, that what the authors term "the process of becoming mind" deconstructs the duality allowing for the notion that creativity – *the making of meaning* – is what moves the developing mind forward and protects it from the risk of inertia, from the accompanying disorder wherein the potential for crisis resides.

I will look *not* at what has been the contextual focus of psychoanalysis since its inception (whatever one's theoretical bias) – the tripartite structure of the psyche (id, ego, and superego) with its conflicts and defenses – but at the imagination's capacity to free the mind by way of its innate curiosity and drive to play, its deriving of pleasure from creative exploration and the giving of form to new ways of seeing and thinking that fulfill the need for and offer the gift of resilience. I will look *not* at the classical notion of sublimation such as it was conceived by Freud, not that it is any less valuable a concept today, but at its enrichment by the interdisciplinary discourse that psychoanalysis has more recently undertaken with neuroscience. For certain innate reflexes, instincts even, may be said to "drive" curiosity, to impel the creative impulse in view of the satisfaction of biological need. Indeed, whether in science or art, the science of art, or the art of science, the relation between curiosity and creativity is complex but certain: Both, in a sense, are driven by a form of crisis, that of *not* knowing; its psychodynamic, neurochemical, and neurobiological consequences; the implicit *need* for knowledge upon which our very existence depends. If we are to uncover the complex processes that, fueled by the integration of nature and nurture, account for the emergence and growth of the mind, if we are to uncover the neural mechanisms and the psychic components that together account for the subjective experience of self and, also, allow for the self's ongoing adaptation to reality, *that* is the arena on which we need now to focus. "Out of the darkness and formlessness something evolves," wrote Wilfred Bion of the analytic session.[38] And it is to *that* evolution of form – how formlessness itself comes to constitute form as seen in the work of a select number of artists – that the pages that follow are devoted. These are artists whose work, when explored in the context of a non-deterministic point of view, fosters reflection on, and even rejection of, variations of the conclusion recently reached by some that an apprehension of self or identification of real-world phenomena are fundamental to aesthetic appeal.

Curiosity is the feature of humankind that leads one to contemplate the kind of change necessitated by the socio-political "viruses" with which we are confronted, the feature that will ultimately liberate us. Sartre's recognition of an elemental freedom of our species and his call to commitment as a moral responsibility remain ever relevant, and if the questions he poses in *What is Literature?* are exceedingly fundamental they are in no way excessively so. They are what invite inquiry into others, questions such as: *Why are humans curious? How does curiosity drive creativity? When might crisis mean, when might it stimulate, and when might it deter that drive?* They are questions that provoke multiple kinds of inquiry that extend from the phenomenological to the metapsychological – or, as Solms has qualified it, the "meta*neuro*psychological"[39] – which is to say never without the neurologic component that renders the brain mindful and mindfulness categorically of the brain. That said, what follows is written with full awareness that "the sciences of the body and the mind," as neuroscientist Shimon Harom has written, "are systematic languages *about* the body, thoughts, and experiences; they are not *the* body nor *the* thoughts or experiences."[40] What follows is also written with full awareness that, as Mark Rothko famously put it, "A painting is not a picture of an experience. It *is* an experience."[41]

Notes

1 Jacques Garelli, "Foreword: Introduction to the Problematic of Gilbert Simondon," in Gilbert Simondon, *Individuation in Light of Notions of Form and Information*, trans. Taylor Adkins (University of Minnesota Press, 2020), xxv.
2 Bruno Latour, *Facing Gaia: Eight Lectures on the New Climatic Regime*, trans. Catherine Porter (Polity Press, 2007), 4.
3 Lois Oppenheim, *A Curious Intimacy: Art and Neuro-psychoanalysis* (Routledge, 2005).
4 Mark Solms, *The Only Cure: Freud and the Neuroscience of Mental Healing* (Weidenfeld & Nicholson, 2026).
5 Joseph Le Doux is another whose work on the neurobiology of affect is also of exceptional importance, but his emphasis lies elsewhere. His perspective on the origin of conscious feelings differs from that of the others whose work is more closely aligned with the focus on aesthetics that is my purpose here.
6 Lisa Feldman Barrett. "Knowledge vs. Creativity." https://iai.tv/video/knowledge-v-creativity?utm_source=YouTube&utm_medium=description

7 Karl Friston, "Computational Psychiatry: From Synapses to Sentience," *Molecular Psychiatry* 28 (2023): 257, 258. doi:10.1038/s41380-022-01743-z
8 Dermot Moran, *Edmund Husserl: The Crisis of the European Sciences and Transcendental Phenomenology: An Introduction* (Cambridge University Press, 2011), 1, 7, 8.
9 Jean-Paul Sartre, *What is Literature*?, trans. Bernard Frechtman (Philosophical Library, 1949), 22.
10 François Noudelmann, "What Do Jean-Paul Sartre and Simone de Beauvoir Have to Say to Us Today?," *Diogenes* 216 (2007): 38.
11 Noudelmann, "What Do Jean-Paul Sartre and Simone de Beauvoir Have to Say to Us Today?," 38 (emphasis added).
12 Cited by Susan Sontag, *Against Interpretation* (Farrar, Straus & Giroux, 1961), 115.
13 Noudelmann, "What Do Jean-Paul Sartre and Simone de Beauvoir Have to Say to Us Today?," 38.
14 François Ansermet and Pierre Magistretti, *The Biology of Freedom: Neural Plasticity, Experience, and the Unconscious* (Other Press, 2007), 183, 192.
15 Alice Jardine, *At the Risk of Thinking* (Bloomsbury, 2020), 4.
16 Noudelmann, "What Do Jean-Paul Sartre and Simone de Beauvoir Have to Say to Us Today?," 38.
17 Garelli, "Foreword: Introduction to the Problematic of Gilbert Simondon," xxv.
18 Garelli, "Foreword: Introduction to the Problematic of Gilbert Simondon," xxvii.
19 Cited by Muriel Combes in *Gilbert Simondon and the Philosophy of the Transindividual*, trans. Thomas LaMarre (MIT Press, 2013), 2.
20 Cited by Combes, *Gilbert Simondon and the Philosophy of the Transindividual*, 7.
21 See Karl Friston and Ivan Herreros, "Active Inference and Learning in the Cerebellum," *Neural Computation* 28 (2016), 1812–39. DOI: 10.1162/NECO_a_00863
22 Sigmund Freud, "The 'Uncanny,'" in *The Standard Edition of the Complete Psychological Works of Sigmund Freud* [hereafter *Standard Edition*], ed. James Strachey, vol. 17, (Hogarth Press, 1955), 244.
23 Jardine, *At the Risk of Thinking*, 238.
24 Volney P. Gay, *Freud on Sublimation* (State University of New York Press, 1992), 13.
25 Jardine, *At the Risk of Thinking*, 11.
26 Cf. Kevin Aho, "The Uncanny in the Time of Pandemics: Heideggerian Reflections on the Coronavirus," *Existential Analysis* 32, no. 1 (January 2021): 5.
27 Moran, *Edmund Husserl: The Crisis of the European Sciences and Transcendental Phenomenology*, 7, 8.
28 Jean-Paul Sartre, *Qu'est-ce que la Littérature*? (Gallimard, 1948), 15 (trans. mine).
29 Sartre, *Qu'est-ce que la Littérature*?, 17.
30 Jacques Garelli, "Il y a le monde," *Esprit* (1982) : 113.
31 Jardine, *At the Risk of Thinking*, 11.
32 Jardine, *At the Risk of Thinking*, 11.
33 Noudelmann, "What Do Jean-Paul Sartre and Simone de Beauvoir Have to Say to Us Today?," 37.
34 Sartre, *Qu'est-ce que la Littérature?*, 27 (trans. mine).
35 Jean-Paul Sartre, *L'Existentialisme est un humanisme* (Les Éditions Nagel, 1946), 47 (trans. mine).
36 Garelli, Foreword: *Introduction to the Problematic of Gilbert Simondon*, xxv.
37 See Mark Solms and Karl Friston, "How and Why Consciousness Arises," *Journal of Consciousness Studies* 25, no. 5–6 (2018): 202–38.
38 Wilfred Bion, "Notes on Memory and Desire," *Psychoanalytic Forum* 2, no. 3 (1967): 272.

39 Mark Solms, "New Project for a Scientific Psychology: General Scheme," *Neuropsychoanalysis* 22 (2020): 5–35. DOI: 10.1080/15294145.2020.1833361
40 Shimon Harom, "Dialogue across Chasm: Are Psychology and Neurophysiology Incompatible?," *Neuron* 107 (August 19, 2020): 601.
41 Cited by Eric Kandel in *Reductionism in Art and Brain Science* (Columbia University Press, 2016), 130 (emphasis added).

Chapter 1

"Becoming Mind"

Sentio ergo sum (I feel therefore I am) might well have been the title of this chapter to be devoted to the meaning of "mind," a concept whose implicit if not explicit investigation would appear preliminary to any consideration of the making and viewing of visual art, preliminary to *creativity* and thereby to *curiosity* and the evasion of *crisis.* Crisis, as we shall see, need not imply catastrophe as such, in the ordinary sense of the word. Rather, aligning with its Greek root meaning to decide, to choose, and its implication of decisive outcome, it may refer to "critical" consequences ensuing from an organism's failure to minimize uncertainty, from the brain's failure to elicit sensorial or behavioral response in accordance with predictions of the future, as Karl Friston and adherents of the self-organizing framework known as "predictive processing" would have it. This capacity to *generate predictions*, to minimize surprise through the integration of perception and affect, and to *generate corrections* to prediction errors is the result of feeling, the result of learning, and the result of their interrelation. And it is the fundamental feeling states and the learning they induce which bring us to the question of just what we mean by "mind" and how it becomes what is, in essence, a *self-generational* system.

Conceptualizing Mind

What is this so-called "mental" engagement with, say, a canvas, this engagement that produces or responds to something aesthetic? How is it related to what we feel in the process? The notion of "mind," in relation both to the physical matter we call "brain" and the immaterial psychic experience of self, is no longer limited by the Cartesian impasse with which the Western world was once confronted and that is so precisely because sentience has come to the fore both in the neurophysiological and psychodynamic domains. Indeed, the many dichotomies that have long characterized philosophical investigations into the phenomenology of mental function – subject/object, internal/external, emotion/cognition, and the like – would appear now to be at the threshold of unification and the basis of that union is feeling. As Susan Sontag, the foremost American

DOI: 10.4324/9781003566755-2

intellectual of the twentieth century, put it, "Thinking is a form of feeling; feeling is a form of thinking."[1] "Becoming Mind," however, was selected as this chapter's title for its emphasis on generativity or emergence: "The mind arises from various biological activities and only gradually assumes the psychological existence that we designate as mind."[2] So begins a nearly 200-page, unpublished manuscript, a book-length draft reporting the results of an observational study whose surtitle is borrowed here. I will return to that manuscript below but the immediate point I would make is this: Philosophy of mind, with its focus on the nature of consciousness and its connection with the body, and developmental psychology, focused on the changes that occur in infancy and childhood (and well beyond) to account for one's sense of who one is, have reached a common ground: the recognition of feeling as the origin of meaning and, thereby, the foundation of consciousness itself. The notion of mind as becoming, as generativity, as emergence by way of prediction and resolution of prediction error, interestingly aligns with much that we associate with modernism (whether deemed high, late, or post) in the literary and visual arts. As has been noted with regard to the writing of Samuel Beckett, for instance, "'becoming' reflects the incessant movement of Beckett's characters, who exist in a perpetual state of liminality," a state typified by "an absence of definitive beginnings or ends. Unlike traditional narratives, which follow a clear trajectory, Beckett's liminal spaces challenge us to rethink the relationship between being and becoming." To that statement by Jonathan Boulter, Asijit Datta (who was interviewing Boulter) replied, "This radical liminality underscores the idea that human experience, as Beckett depicts it, is marked by an absence of signposts or certainties, reflecting the haunting quality of existence itself. Thus, Beckett offers [...] an invitation to engage with the complexities of subjectivity in a world stripped of clear definitions and boundaries."[3] What might that engagement mean? How might it reflect what occurs in aesthetic experience generally speaking or in the modernist endeavor more specifically?

In 2019, consciousness was proclaimed by physicist Paul Davies the "number-one problem of science, of existence even."[4] David Chalmers, a philosopher and neural scientist, had already, some two and a half decades prior, famously termed the subjective nature of the physiology of neurons the "hard problem," going so far as to say "The really hard problem of consciousness is the problem of *experience*."[5] But what does *that* mean? And how do we get from that question to feeling and its coming to light as the unifying factor of the multiple schisms characteristic of Western thought since, at least, Antiquity? What, moreover, does any of that have to do with curiosity and creativity, as in the making of visual and literary art, and what has crisis to do with any of it? My objective is not to delve deeply either into the neuroscience or the philosophy of mind. Consideration of how consciousness arises and why we experience what we do is best left to the neuroscientists, neuropsychologists, and others. Yet particularly pertinent to the aim of this book – to investigating the making of meaning, the meaning of making/

viewing visual art, and the implicit relation to crisis that lies, as we shall see, therein – is where they meet, for it is there – in *feeling*, as noted above – that the "hard problem" not only becomes resolvable but bears significantly on the three topics at hand – curiosity, creativity, and crisis – and their interrelation. Indeed, *feeling integrates emotion, memory, and meaning, the primordial components of art, and it does so for artist and viewer alike.*

Suffice it to say, therefore, that the "hard problem of consciousness," unlike the "easy problems of consciousness" from which Chalmers clearly distinguishes it, is so called, as one would expect, because of the difficulty of explanation. A number of phenomena that we associate with consciousness are explainable by neuropsychological or neurophysiological means. Or, if they are not fully explainable, at least the direction that needs to be taken to move closer to their explication is identifiable. Examples of such phenomena, the "easy problems," include for Chalmers "the ability to discriminate, categorize, and react to environmental stimuli," "the reportability of mental states," "the focus of attention," and so on.[6] Conversely, the so-called "hard problem" is difficult insofar as its very reason for being is not detectable. "Why is it," he asks, "that when our cognitive systems engage in visual and auditory information-processing, we have visual or auditory experience: the quality of deep blue, the sensation of middle C?" And, he inquires, "It is widely agreed that experience arises from a physical basis, but we have no good explanation of why and how it so arises. Why should physical processing give rise to a rich inner life at all?"[7]

Neuropsychologist and psychoanalyst Mark Solms has further defined the problem by referencing Sir Francis Crick, the molecular biologist who, with James Watson and Rosalind Franklin, discovered the structure of DNA. Crick believed in the physical basis of experience and, while Chalmers did not disagree, he was insistent that any explanation for this basis was lacking. Though Crick, and the cognitive neuroscience to which his belief gave rise, insisted that "the vast assembly of nerve cells and their associated molecules" were the basis of conscious experience, identifying (as he and others did and would continue to do) "the specific brain processes that *correlate* with experience," just how these correlates were responsible for *causing* experience was not described. As Solms put the question: "That is the hard part of the problem: how and why do neurophysiological activities *produce* the experience of consciousness? In other words, how does matter *become* mind?"[8]

Notwithstanding the complexity of the question, I will consider in what follows two approaches to it, not so much the question as two ways it has been investigated: The first an observational child development study undertaken some sixty-odd years ago; the second an amalgam of scientific inquiries informed by neuroscience, psychoanalysis, and their interconnection in what has come to be known as neuropsychoanalysis. What I hope to make clear is *the convergence in feeling* of the insights obtained and, in subsequent chapters, the import of that convergence in the aesthetic domain, its relevance, once again, to curiosity, creativity, and crisis as well.

A Prospective Observational Approach

In the 1960s, a highly esteemed psychiatrist and psychoanalyst, Dr. Peter Neubauer, determined that the policy of a New York City adoption agency to separate identical twins and place them in different homes offered a unique research opportunity: the possibility of studying prospectively, as opposed to retrospectively (as had previously been done), identical twins raised apart. Though it is generally assumed that no written account of the results was produced, the research team, consisting of Drs. Samuel Abrams and Christa Balzert, in addition to Neubauer, did, in fact, produce not only several papers[9] but this exceedingly comprehensive and illuminating draft dating to the early '90s which the authors decided for reasons of confidentiality not to put into print. The title of this chapter bears part of that manuscript's name, whose full title is "Becoming Mind: Identical Twins Reared Apart," precisely because the focus of that work, from which much is to be learned, is the meaning of "I" and how it becomes what it is; in short, the mind itself.

The study, commonly known as "The Neubauer Twins Study," has stimulated a number of difficult questions ranging from the psychological impact of separating multiples put up for adoption to the ethics of research involving adoptive families who knew virtually nothing of the study in which they were participating. The proliferation of errors pertaining to the circumstances and the basis for the decision to separate render these questions even more complex.[10] At issue as well is how one views today the practices of a bygone era: Do we consider them in accordance with the standards maintained at the time or with the standards developed many years later? (The Institutional Review Board was not established until 1974; the Belmont Report dates to 1978.)[11] None of this, however, is germane to what I wish to make known here, the principal findings of this prospective observational study pertaining to the "complex process of *becoming* mind."[12]

Indeed, entirely independent of any such issues the unique situation provided the observational team by the rearing of monozygotic (or identical) twins apart is revealed in the unpublished book: "Monozygotic twins are endowed with a common genetic pool. They provide an opportunity to isolate the dispositional factors that influence the move from a globally biological organ system to a differentiated mind." Whereas such twins reared together "share nurture as well as nature," with the result that "explanations intended to account for the sources of similarities or differences between them cannot be neatly sorted out into the one or the other category," when "different settings" provide the locus for the activation of "the same inherent potential," the "contributions from nature and nurture can be isolated more readily."

The goals of the study included, therefore, in addition to studying matters relating to adoption and, potentially, the notions of abnormality and normality, "the growth of the mind," how "becoming mind" involves the extraction of "formative experiences from the yield of disposition and the environment." That, in a word, was the primary objective. This essential purpose was further detailed by Balzert in a subsequent paper. What she, along with Neubauer and Abrams, was seeking to uncover were answers to the following: "Can our premise of a maturational blueprint that underlies a child's development be validated? Are there instances where the developmental pull forward is so compromised as to assure a disordered development independent from the environmental offerings? Which are the environmental conditions that are capable of derailing an otherwise intact underlying blueprint? Can an adequate environment compensate for an otherwise compromised blueprint or alter the program that influences the style of development and the phase dominance?"

Balzert also wrote, however, of the "[m]arked differences in parental personalities and attitudes" that were shown to make no difference whatsoever in development, further illustrating the error of the mind-brain duality.[13] While understanding psychopathology was not the goal – rather, it was "the emergence of mind from the underlying biological activities that sponsor its growth" – findings of the observations over the ten- to twelve-year period in which the study took place did cause the authors, as noted in the introduction, "to view some aspects of psychopathology in a way quite different than [their] antecedent frames of reference could have provided." In fact, in elucidating the relationship between nature and nurture, the team, Balzert wrote in "Genetic Findings and Their Impact on the Psychoanalytic Theory of Development," was more impressed with the likenesses than the dissimilarities between particular siblings, "with the fundamental similarities ... found in spite of significant differences in environmental offerings." As Balzert said, "I can only hint [at] the excitement and occasional distress all of us experienced when our data challenged some of our longheld beliefs about human development and the origins of pathology."[14] The notion of "disposition" as integral to development and the idea that dispositional features, in interacting with the environment, may not only be determinative of psychic development but, also, of clinical disorders, were both incidental and highly significant.

"If children share a common biological heritage and the surround is so important for development, one would imagine that substantive differences in the environment would inevitably yield substantive differences in outcome," wrote Abrams regarding the results of the study. But there were monozygotic siblings who "turned out to be remarkably similar at every step in the study and at the end of the formal period of the study as well. Their differences were merely stylistic, not substantive, or they were accountable on the basis of other factors such as congenital influences. The hypothesis was proposed that an inherent component was at work, one that arose early and exerted a continuing effect upon development as growth went on." And, indeed, this hypothesis – the supposition that "normal development proceeds in an expectable sequence of progressive hierarchical organizations in accord with a biological blueprint and driven by an inherent impetus" – was substantiated along with what the team would come to consider a disorder, one attributable not to neurotic conflict but to an impairment in the "forward pull," to a deficit in the "inherent impetus."[15] This "new disorder," as described by the team, manifests in the paucity of organizational sequences and in "limitations in the forward movement in affectivity, cognition, and behavior, resulting in a clinical picture of quite serious and somewhat discoordinate immaturity." This deficiency in "forward pull" was a finding that the team, already at that time, determined of benefit to clinical psychiatry and psychoanalysis to the extent that "the presence of an adequate forward pull" has bearing on assessment of behavior and recommendations for treatment.

More to the point, however, is that the nature vs. nurture formulation itself, a dichotomy that continues to inspire debate among theorists today – though in more complex neuroscientific, neurophilosophical, and neuropsychoanalytic articulations – is a formulation that remains the basis of much assumptive thinking on the part of the public at large and thereby the basis of much of the stigma surrounding mental disorders as well. Yet it was utterly deconstructed by the study, leading the authors of the manuscript to conclude:

> The environment's competence can only be comprehended in terms of the specific inherent capacities and limitations of children; this attends to the reciprocal interaction between the components of the equation rather than either in isolation. This also shifts the focus of attention away from "nature vs nurture" to the process of becoming mind and to the necessary experiential products.
>
> This recognition of the mutual interdependence of disposition and the environment seems to provide a more felicitous framework for understanding the process of becoming mind than does any approach that isolates the one from the other or sees one as more "causative" than the other.

While it is *the mind's relation to the neurophysiology of the brain and its constitution as a non-physical entity* that is the preliminary subject at hand (preliminary to the relation of consciousness to curiosity and creativity in aesthetics and to the potential for avoidance of crisis therein), it is in *the deconstruction of the nature vs. nurture juxtaposition* that the significance of the study itself resides. And it is precisely this deconstruction by way of observation – this deconstruction with its concomitant integration of biological givens and psychosocial contextualizations – that is affirmed by the neuropsychoanalytic theorization to which we will shortly turn.

Over the course of the prospective study of four sets of monozygotic twins reared apart, "becoming mind" came to be understood by the authors in terms of three distinct categories according to which their observations could be described: "the matured functions which continuously shape and mold, the emerging discontinuities which are being pulled forward, and the actions of assembly of these static and dynamic constituents." To put it otherwise, the authors' insights into the emergence (in the sense of continual becoming) of mind came to be viewed in accordance with a continual assembling of elements already well-developed with those yet progressing, those responding to the forward pull of development. And what the team came to see was the extent to which "constitutional givens" delimit "what can be extracted from the environment to become formative mental experience." "Becoming mind" was explained, then, as a developmental sequence extending from the world of the infant, "*a world founded in biology*," to a world "*constructed from meanings*."[16]

In a word, the three categories that frame the process of "becoming mind" – "continuities, discontinuities, and assembly" – were shown to be far more significantly impacted by what the authors refer to as the "inherent (or dispositional) *equipment*" of the individual than anticipated. With regard to continuities and discontinuities, Drs. Neubauer, Abrams, and Balzert differentiate between a coterie of functions apparent early in the developmental process, often influencing it, and other functions that emerge later and are dependent upon still other "emerging discontinuous hierarchies" or "environmental interactions." The earlier manifesting functions, moreover, were found not only to shape "what was destined to occur," but to be unmodified by later growth. Among them, and intimately linked to – indeed, deeply implanted within – this "inherent (or dispositional) equipment" is *affect*.

The expression of affect (situated by the authors within the psychological arena of the ego) is indisputably determined by interaction with the environment. Confirmed by observation, this interaction, however, was overshadowed by the finding that the "inherent equipment" plays a far greater role in the actual shaping of certain elements of affect than is generally assumed. Moreover, as revealed in the manuscript, affect came to be seen by the authors not only as inherently equipmental, which is to say indicative of "early expressions of biology" or dispositional, but as itself impacting the environment: "More precisely, the maturation of id and ego and their mutual influence shape affect development. From the standpoint of the drives, the intensity and balance of libidinal and aggressive instincts impact upon total affective expression. However, features of the ego and of the developmental progression also influence the drive-environmental interplay, thereby modifying the final nature of the affect products." The authors were completely convinced as a result of their study that both "intensity and modulation of affect are inherent givens" and almost as convinced that the same is to be said of what they call the "range and orchestration" of affect as well. (It is to be noted that "inherent givens" refers not only to the genetic pool passed on from one generation to another, but also to congenital inherence.)

An "equipmental continuity," affect is defined by the authors as "a sustained feeling or emotional tone that characterizes an individual." Additionally, affect is regarded by them "as a superordinate division under which mood and specific emotions are subsumed." Descriptively speaking, we are told that "affect is like music, assessed in terms of its range (the breadth or repertoire of emotional expression), intensity (the degree of feeling), orchestration (the assembly and the harmony), modulation (the regulation or the toning up or down of emotions), the degree of differentiation of the discrete emotions, and characteristic abiding mood." And, conceptually speaking,

> the maturation of id and ego and their mutual influence shape affect development. From the standpoint of the drives, the intensity and balance of libidinal and aggressive instincts impact upon total affective expression. However, features of the ego and of the developmental progression also influence the drive-environmental interplay, thereby modifying the final nature of the affect products. The expression of discrete emotions is part of the ego's repertoire. New organizations of affect-experiences and discrete emotions emerge at different levels of development, reflecting the integrative tendencies of the ego and the evolving transformational capacities of the developmental progression. Thus, the progressive differentiation of affect experiences is dependent upon the integrity of the overall developmental process as well as the growth of the ego and id. Consequently, from a conceptual point of view, it is not always easy to separate the varying intra- and inter-systemic features that underlie the phenomenologic aspects of affect that are readily observable.

If I cite at some length the authors' understanding of affect, it is due precisely to the importance given the determination of some, if not many, affective features by the "inherent equipment." It is due to the primacy of affect, its embeddedness in human experience. Negative vs. positive tone (or "abiding mood"), for instance, was found to be more clustered around birth order, degrees of sinistrality, or other constituents of the inherent, albeit congenital, equipment. Resistant to this finding, insofar as it counters "the conventional wisdom that regards affect as so much more pliable," which is to say so much more "determined by external influences," the authors nonetheless were obliged to accept as "inherent givens" not only the intensity of affect, but its modulation as well and the idea that both range and orchestration are highly likely to be of the same order. The point, moreover, is that the findings regarding affect support the broader view of the emergence of mind; that is, the broader view of development as *the very emergence of consciousness, the self-organization dependent upon the valence of feeling*. "Development occurs in a sequence of phase-dominated plateaus, each hierarchically ordered. The pattern or style of phase emergence is determined by components of the inherent maturationally-determined program [...]. The program introduces potential new ways of being, thinking and acting, a potential that is actualized by way of interactions with specific (and variable) nutrients in the surround. The interaction results in experiences, which become nodal points for newly evolving structures." Consider, for example, a set of twins exhibiting similar expressions of a shared "poorly organized and persistent" developmental phase, "poor differentiation and little evidence of reorganization into new hierarchies." They experience at precisely the same age fears "not of phobic origin, i.e., not based in internal conflicts," but the result of impairment in the "evolvement of age-appropriate internalized object representations."

The "becoming" of mind, in sum, was found by the authors to consist in a developmental organization extending, as noted above, from "a world founded in biology to one constructed from meanings." I will return to the significance of *meaning* for "becoming mind," to the notion of the affective emergence of mind from matter or the physicality of the brain and the cognitive impact upon the forward drive, what impels the mind to be what it is. First, however, a brief look at the recent findings of another, very different approach to the study of mind as an emergent of brain and how it relates to the findings put forth in *Becoming Mind: Identical Twins Reared Apart.*

The Neuropsychoanalytic Perspective

Mark Solms, from whose work in neuropsychology and psychoanalysis the discipline of neuropsychoanalysis came into being, has demonstrated with regard to the "hard problem" – the emanation of mind from matter / psyche from brain – that consciousness, or mindfulness, *is* by its very nature *the state of being subjective*: Absent subjectivity, absent an experiencing subject, Solms tells us, there is no awareness of the cognitive representations, or mental objects, that distinguish the "mental" from the "real." And the primary modality of the "mental" – of the mind to which experience, and thereby subjectivity, is requisite – is affect, which is pre-reflexive and present from birth.[17]

Insofar as consciousness is innately affective, its foremost function is neither to perceive nor comprehend, but to feel. Feelings, in fact, actually "*do* something" in being mindful: They serve our chances of survival. It is the affective modality of consciousness that bears witness to the visceral states of the body that ensure its homeostatic equilibrium, as Solms, Jaak Panksepp, Antonio Damasio, and others have shown. Simply put, it takes both feeling and, consequently, knowing how we are feeling to keep ourselves alive. Neuropsychoanalysis builds upon this premise, upon the Freudian view of affect as key to understanding the concept of mind to the extent that it is foundational feeling states – with Solms substituting satiation for Freud's notion of pleasure – that inform us of how adequately our biological needs and drives are being met. It almost goes without saying that there are multiple connotations of affect in its relation to emotion, just as there are many ways of thinking about drive in relation to instinct and other such notions key to neuroscience and psychoanalysis alike. But the point is that neuropsychoanalysis, in distinguishing between the demands made by the mind and the actuality of the responses to those demands, reveals just how complex is the idea of development. And, in favoring the subjectivity of feeling as a state of being upon which consciousness depends, while also attending to the objective and thus observable and measurable workings of mentation, neuropsychoanalysis *reveals as a false dichotomy the division of nature and nurture, a schism endlessly perpetuated, however discretely, by the "hard problem" (as a split between mind and matter) itself.*

As Solms and Margaret Zellner have explained,

> Because the internal states themselves cannot be objectively measured, [some cognitive neuroscientists] focus [...] on external observables such as emotional stimuli and responses – *behaviours* – or other objective *correlates* of emotions such as physiological changes. We believe that this is where the big differences between the psychoanalytic and or scientific perspectives on affect arise. For psychoanalysts, feelings in and of themselves have causal consequences.[18]

Part and parcel of neuroscientific and psychoanalytic consideration alike, feelings are deemed by Solms and Zellner as really in existence, as "really a part of nature." "[T]he subjective aspect of the mind is there for good biological reasons," they submit, reasons that merit explaining as much as any others.[19]

Similarly, Jaak Panksepp, in illuminating foundational emotional (as differentiated from bodily) systems, systems said to constitute the affective groundwork for the higher realms of what Freud called the "mental apparatus," approached from a scientific stance the neural infrastructure of affective experience. In a paper entitled "A meditation on the affective neuroscientific view of human and animalian brains," Panksepp, along with co-author Lucy Biven, explains how affect and raw emotional expression may be related. To do so, they adopt a dual-aspect monist perspective: "*Monism*, as opposed to mind/body *dualism*, means that all emotional expressions and feelings can be traced back to the stuff of the brain. The *dual aspect* refers to the two facets of emotional expression: affective feelings and emotional actions/behaviours. This means that when any emotional system is aroused, people and animals have two responses: they experience an affect and they are motivated to behave in particular ways."[20]

So, too, Solms makes eminently clear in his writings that it is a dual-aspect monist view that allows for resolution of the "hard problem," that it is a dual-aspect monist perspective that accounts for the inherently affective, experientially subjective, foundational states of consciousness, on the one hand, and for the higher order of consciousness, on the other, wherein cognitive and perceptual representational objects reside. That is to say that it is in terms of the neurophysiological mechanisms of the brain that the mind is to be understood, that it is in responding to these mechanisms (whether reflexively, behaviorally, or otherwise) that consciousness, as the experience of awareness (conscious or not), occurs. Thus, there are two ways of approaching the single or monist phenomenon that is mind: one observational, whether data-based as in the Neubauer study or via the imaging of neural structures and related functions of the brain; the other seeking insight into the feelings associated with them. And it is here that the authors of the *Becoming Mind* manuscript and theorists of neuropsychoanalysis meet.

The Neubauer, Abrams, Balzert manuscript, in proposing the "continuities, discontinuities and assembly" model of the emergent mind, looks upon the mental from both the subjective and objective points of view to account for the co-existence of continuous and discontinuous growth, to account for "functions already formed and enlarging and those still requiring progressive differentiation and transformation." It regards the mind from the dual-aspect monist perspective to account for the fueling and constraining that disposition and the environment impose upon it in the service of stability and survival. And it underscores the biologically determined "pull forward" that allows for the progression of the individual through the phases of development. It is when that seemingly magnetic draw forward, that pull in accordance with its biological blueprint, is rendered deficient that instability or dysregulation occurs. *As such, it is the mind, as both object and subject, that the manuscript authors address; in other words, feelings as regulators of the reflexive process to which experience gives rise.*

Such is the dual-aspect monist perspective to which neuropsychoanalysis similarly subscribes. And it is this perspective that affords resolution of the "hard problem," that elucidates how a corporeal phenomenon is at once the non-corporeal phenomenon that is mind, allowing for an understanding of feeling as the *sine qua non* of what is now often referred to as the MindBrain. Neuropsychoanalysis, in fact, is based upon the dual-aspect monist approach that Freud himself already favored, the approach that considers the mind, in itself epistemologically unknowable, in actuality unconscious and generative of reflexive or conscious awareness.[21] Solms' approach to "the hard problem" offers a view of consciousness that differentiates between "the *subject* of consciousness and *objects* of consciousness" while retaining the singleness of the conscious modality of being. "Objects of consciousness," he has explained, are necessarily perceived by a conscious, which is to say experiencing, subject. With the cessation of consciousness, "objects of consciousness" exist no longer. In providing the key to unlocking the problem of how matter (the brain) becomes (the non-material) mind, Solms relies on the notion that cognitive representations are not the locus of consciousness nor its mode of being insofar as such representations – or "mental solids (objects)" – are fundamentally experiential. In a word, the primary modality of awareness lies elsewhere. And where the modality of awareness resides, as Solms has persuasively argued, is in *affect*.[22]

Solms has published widely on the dual-aspect monist perspective. But it is his radical revision of Sigmund Freud's *Project for a Scientific Psychology*[23] that perhaps best illustrates the fundamentally erroneous nature of the dichotomies characterizing the presumed phenomenology of mental function – subject/object, internal/external, emotion/cognition, and so on.

Rendering metapsychology a "meta*neuro*psychology," as he calls it, he creates a natural science of psychology, the study of mind, and effectively resolves, or at least nears resolution of, the Chalmers conundrum. As he explains in the introduction to his line-by-line updating of Freud's work, the "'Project for a Scientific Psychology' is the Rosetta Stone of neuropsychoanalysis. It was the foundational text for the whole of what became known as metapsychology – Freud's basic theory of the functional dynamics of the mind – *and* a sophisticated model of the neural mechanisms by which those dynamics come about. In other words, the 'Project' (as it came to be abbreviated) was the first attempt – Freud's own attempt – to achieve what the whole interdisciplinary endeavor called neuropsychoanalysis is trying to achieve today."[24]

Neuropsychoanalysis is increasingly coming to be accepted by those who have long maintained a more stringently classical (or Freudian) perspective on clinical work as well as by others whose orientation is less ego psychological. In addition to reducing tensions between psychoanalytic orientations, it is diminishing conceptual differences between disciplines, psychoanalysis and neuroscience most obviously, but also psychoanalysis and physics, psychoanalysis and philosophy, and psychoanalysis and art, as we shall see through the course of this book. Nonetheless, I would offer this caveat: I would contend that there are terms whose inconsistent usage by both neuropsychoanalysts and neuroscientists (affective and cognitive alike) impedes an even wider appreciation of *feeling as the key to resolving "the hard problem"* and impedes, as a result, apprehension of the dual-aspect monist perspective as the key to deconstructing the mind/body and nature/nurture dichotomies. The ontology of experience – the "I" that feels and then reflects[25] – will not be fully apprehended until these terms are rethought and consistency of their usage is obtained.

The Linguistic Quagmire and Why It Matters

To cite but three examples, there is the word "conscious" itself. Most often, it is used synonymously with the state of wakefulness: A person is said to be conscious if awake and responsive. Of course, there are degrees of consciousness as determined neurologically, but clearly the implication of being conscious is that one is not asleep or in a vegetative state or coma. Initially, Freud descriptively considered consciousness in the context of a mental system. He was later to view it not as a system, but a quality pertaining to the psyche, whether a feature of affect, fantasy, or objects of perception external to the mind.[26] Considering it dynamically, he clearly decried "abuse of the word 'conscious,'" objecting to the notion of an "unconscious consciousness" and distinguishing between preconscious (or "foreconscious") and unconscious, the former able to pass into consciousness easily, the latter unable to do so as detached from consciousness.[27]

But here's the rub: If awake and responsive signifies being conscious, is one who is not in such a state "unconscious"? Alternatively, is one not conscious to be deemed "nonconscious," a word no less ambiguous? As I have shown elsewhere,[28] "nonconscious" is a widely used term; it is, in fact, a defining term of much current research insofar as "conscious" has meaning only in relation to "nonconscious" mental function. But neither is used with the consistency required for the kind of interdisciplinary dialogue increasingly needed for a deeper understanding of the mind, what it both experiences and produces. The semantic entanglement, the inconsistent usage of "unconscious" vs. "nonconscious" in the literature, poses challenges at once structural and hermeneutic, by which is meant challenges with regard to our understanding of psychic organization and the interpretation of meaning made by the mind. It poses challenges, in a word, to our understanding of what it is to be conscious, to our understanding of the mind itself.

A second example is to be found in the use of the word "intentionality." A notion studied since antiquity, its use today is very variable. Freud conceived of intentionality in the sense not only of conscious volition but unconscious motivation as well, while for Husserl the term played a significantly more expansive role in both thought and experience. Franz Brentano (with whom both Freud and Husserl studied and who took issue with Husserl's transformation of the term into what Quentin Lauer called "an a priori idealism"[29]) used intentionality to mean object-orientation, whether the object existed inside or outside the mind. Phenomenologists – Martin Heidegger and Maurice Merleau-Ponty most notably and Jacques Garelli more recently – have focused extensively on the spatiotemporal constitution, the "worldifying" experience, that is perception and on intentionality in that context, in the context of the self's orientation toward the object (reflecting the origin of the word "intention" meaning "directed at" in Latin) and self-object unification. Paul Ricoeur wrote of the "invincible unawareness of self that characterizes intentionality in act," an anoetic "bursting forth from self,"[30] while Vittorio Gallese refers to intentionality as "aboutness," as in "the aboutness of our relation to the world,"[31] as had Brentano himself and as does Solms. Solms also speaks of intentionality more specifically in terms of emotional or affective responsiveness to homeostatic need and of the intentionality of "voluntary movements of the other," their being "mirrored in our own premotor neurons," and intentionality being "thereby reproduced in us (i.e., in our own brains)."[32] Solms comments as well on the absence of subjective intentionality in works of art, about which more later. It is his work, alongside that of certain of his contemporaries (Karl Friston and Jaak Pankesepp, in particular), that has extended the boundaries of philosophy, psychology, and neuroscience in such a way as to engage each discipline with the others. But the point is that differing usages of intentionality abound rendering the "hard problem" more complex.

Comparability, as expressed by the notion of "something it is like" – as first Thomas Nagel (in 1974) and some twenty years later Chalmers (in 1995) spoke of it – offers yet a third example. "[A]n organism is conscious," Nagel claimed, "if and only if there is something it is like to be that organism."[33] That, for both philosophers, defined the subjective nature of experience, the subjectivity that *is* experience. Emphasizing "the something-it-is-like-ness of subjective experience,"[34] as Solms refers to it, Nagel, in his celebrated paper "What Is It Like to Be a Bat?," proclaimed the knowledge of a subjective perspective ultimately accessible not merely to a lone individual but to a collective point of view: "At present we are completely unequipped to think about the subjective character of experience without relying on the imagination – without taking up the point of view of the experiential subject." Such was the challenge Nagel proclaimed lay before us, the "challenge to form new concepts and devise a new method – an objective phenomenology not dependent on empathy or the imagination. Though presumably it would not capture everything, its goal would be to describe, at least in part, the subjective character of experiences in a form comprehensible to beings incapable of having those experiences."[35]

What it "feels like" is the buzzword that justifies the primordial position of affect in our understanding of mind. But if affect is the source of sentience and sentience the foundation of consciousness, how can it "feel like" anything but what it is? The notion bespeaks comparability and hence a duality where there is none. I am reminded here of James Joyce's notion of "almosting": "Remember. Haroun al Rashid. I am almosting it. That man led me, spoke."[36] Like "almosting," a derivative of the (non-existent) verb "to almost," "feels like" suffers from the insertion of a fault in the structure of affect. Like the Proustian remembrance of times past, the sensory memory that brings back, however briefly, the feeling of *then*, there is a spatiotemporal split in "feels like" rendering consciousness at a remove from what it is.

When mental processes are considered from a subjective perspective, as opposed to an objective point of view, we say that this is what they feel like. But does "the something-it-is-like-ness of subjective experience" really mean what we wish it to mean? Do we not rather mean that this is *how* it feels? Does it *feel like* something to be awake? To be conscious? If one were to say "This looks like the way to the university," there is no implication of a duality. But "Ms. V. feels like" is meant to relay *how* she feels by the introduction of a metaphor, an inherent schism. And when the "something it is like" is related to feeling, which is to say to subjectivity and thereby lived experience – when how something felt is re-presented as something "out there" – it fails. "Imagine what that feels like," one readily says. But does one feel *like* that? Does a bat feel *like* a bat? Or is the subjective perspective not so subjective when the analogous perspective is introduced, separating the *how it is* from *what it re-presents*? Interestingly, the title of the French translation of Nagel's paper unequivocally drives home the point: "Quel effet cela fait-il d'être une chauve-souris?" ("How does it feel to be a bat?")

But why does it matter? It matters because it is reductive and even erroneous to consider subjectivity and the phenomenology of emotion in terms of comparison, which is to say in terms of something other than what it is. When the "*experience* of consciousness" is said to be "about *what it is like* to perceive or remember,"[37] for instance, one is no closer to knowing about consciousness but something else, something to which it is comparable. Phenomenologically speaking, which is the only way of addressing the issue, one fails as one "undercuts the intrinsic connection between affective, sensory, or bodily, on the one hand, and intentional or evaluative components in emotions' affective intentionality, on the other," to cite Thomas Szanto and Hilge Landweer.[38] Indeed, were feeling – the foundation of consciousness – unrelated to cognition (however pre-reflexive or unthought) and more, it would not exist in the service of homeostasis, the regulation of bodily need, which is precisely what feeling serves, as Solms, Panksepp, Damasio, and others have unmistakably shown.[39]

It matters because a collective understanding of subjective experience is not only in some measure empathic, but reliant on what Sidney Feshbach called the "metamorphic power of the metaphor."[40] I cannot truly understand – which is to say "feel" – your experience as though it were my own and the "*something-it-is*-like-*ness*" impedes our recognition of that. What it is *like* to understand how you felt when something was said to you is not *to know* intrinsically or *to feel* what you felt, for existentially it is not *like* anything else; it is *how it is*. Such is the meaning of subjectivity. Objectivity lies elsewhere. And the linguistic foil impedes our grasp of the necessity and value of the two perspectives. It interferes with our understanding of the meaning of empathy as the attribution of affect by one subject to another and it impedes our grasp of the significance of investigating consciousness, a unitary or monistic phenomenon, from both the subjective and objective points of view.

Thomas Ogden has shown this to be so in his exploration of analytic writing. No clinical illustration of an analyst's experience with a patient *is* the experience; rather, Ogden argues, it is a fiction. However articulate a writer, the analyst, in their effort to convey what transpired, imagines the session: "The patient presented in an analytic paper [...] is not the person lying on the analyst's couch, but an imaginary patient, a fiction, invented in the medium of words, just as a portrait painter creates a work of art, a fiction, an entity in its own right, separate from the person posing for the portrait." Indeed, art, as we shall see, is the perfect illustration (literately and figuratively) of precisely this point. *Nothing created by the mind is reducible to anything pre-existing that expression; rather, for both analyst and patient – as for artist and viewer (or writer and reader, as the case may be) – there is the affective memory association to a prereflexive or nonthetic arena, an ontological arena that is, in a word, irreproducible.* This may well appear nothing short of self-evident, but how often it is forgotten. As Ogden reminds us, even our models of the mind are mere metaphors, objectified metaphorical ideas about which we create stories: "There is no such thing as an ego or a superego [...]. There isn't even an internal world – inside what? Inside our head? Between our ears? We are continually making up stories about 'the mental apparatus' – and, too often, we believe our stories. We forget that we are creating metaphors, writing fiction."[41] So it is that Emil Benveniste could rightly claim, "Ego est qui *dit* ego."

It matters because, as Bruno Clément has articulated the aporic postulate underlying the philosophy of Henri Bergson, "only language is able to save us from language."[42] Recognition of the linguistic quagmire is necessitated by any attempt at resolution of the extraordinary challenge posed by Chalmers: the challenge to locate a perspective at once independent of imagination and empathy and, more exigent still, a perspective that defies the disparity between subjective and objective. Steering clear of the paradigmatic inconsistencies (and even falsities) such as those exemplified in the semantic entanglements noted above, one is led to an approach to "the hard problem" that values the objective and subjective viewpoints in recognizing the value bestowed on each by the other and their relation to the foundation of each. Such is the dual-aspect monist position as upheld by Solms and others.

But why begin a book devoted to neuroaesthetics – to the interplay between curiosity, creativity, and crisis that lies therein – and to the neuropsychoanalytic contextualization of aesthetic experience with an emphatic if cursory mention of the dual-aspect monist perspective? Because this perspective offers a stunning delineation of the MindBrain infrastructure, its development and its vulnerabilities, and in doing so it takes us well beyond the dichotomous paradigms referred to earlier which continually leave us stumped. Because this perspective evades deterministic assumptions regarding the brain in favor of the creative capacity owing to neuronal plasticity, in favor of imagination motivated by curiosity, in favor of the dialectic that sheds light on our sensory experience, our expectations (both interoceptive, produced within our physical beings, and exteroceptive, produced externally), and the potential for crisis when disorder, the lack of predictability, holds sway. Because dual-aspect monism provides insight into the making of meaning and into the value of learning, which is where, as we shall come to see, art and science meet. And because the imaginative and the real are no more oppositional in aesthetic experience than the body and the mind, as it will be my purpose to show. *We know from epigenetics that life experience can alter the expression of some genes leaving the DNA intact, as the observational twins study reveals and the neuropsychoanalytic view of the MindBrain confirms. Similarly, consideration of aesthetic experience, no matter how abstract the work of art, requires recognition of the concordance of emotional drives with the neuronal arousal involved in the creation or apperception of the artwork, the relational dimension at play in the work that constitutes its very ontology.*

From Dialectical Determinism to Subjective Experience

The "emergence of mind from the underlying biological activities that sponsor its growth" was the focus of the Neubauer, Abrams, and Balzert book-in-progress. "Over time we could observe this evolving structure move away from the primary influence of biological activities and toward the dominance of psychological meanings," wrote the authors of the manuscript, where what is achieved is a shift from the nature/nurture schism of causation to the experiential mode of "becoming." Normally, a child "continues to attribute more sophisticated meanings to the stimuli in the surround," notes Abrams in a paper about the findings of the study. Development progresses according to the "readiness of the child to make use of such dressed-up meanings in a facilitating or injurious way," a readiness that "rests to a considerable degree on the inherent competence of the underlying process that guides the emerging phases. That process, fashioned by its inherent impetus and blueprint, is central to the inevitable progressive recycling of meanings," in other words, contextualization.[43] The Neubauer, Abrams, and Balzert manuscript lays bare the discovery, the "becoming" that occurs by way of a "pull forward" toward the making and maturation of mind, and of a "new disorder" defined by an impairment of impetus. "The Process of Becoming Mind" demonstrates just how that forward pull is in the service of a "mental apparatus" whose function it is to reflect and thereby act upon the affect experienced by every human being from birth.

The observational study resulted in a manuscript that reveals, then, how structural entities – "ego, id, superego, ego-ideal and subordinate less complex [structures] like the self-representation, selfobjects, and the collective representation of people and things" – relate to the empirical domain of psychic functions, to "cognition, affectivity, perception, the capacity for representation, the construction of reality, synthesis, and the ability to discriminate dangers and opportunities" – those entities whose very survival depends upon their being "useful." Conceptually framed in accordance with three categories – "matured functions which continuously shape and mold," "emerging discontinuities which are being pulled forward," and "actions of assembly of these static and dynamic constituents" – their observations led to the placement of some dispositional equipment within one or another psychological domain, or within a bridging function between them, and, in the case of other such equipment, where such placement was seemingly unviable, description alone prevailed. Yet, while continuities, discontinuities, and assembly provided organizational categories for the elucidation of the emergence of mind, what became apparent to the team was just how significantly the inherent equipment impacted all three.

Neuropsychoanalysis may be said to provide scientific support for the findings of the observational study as related in the manuscript: With recognition of the value of the dual-aspect monist perspective, what Solms, for one, discloses, as do the authors of the unpublished manuscript, is that consciousness, the advent of awareness or the becoming of mind – *to be understood not as emanating from nothing, but from the subjectivity of feeling* – resides neither solely in cognition (as held by the Enlightenment forebears of cognitive neuroscience and their descendants) nor in perception alone, but in the experience of sentience itself. The observational study of Neubauer, Abrams, and Balzert, the study that dates to the 1960s and produced some three decades later an unpublished manuscript of considerable significance, already uncovered, albeit in preliminary form, *the very integration of the "mental apparatus" with the physical counterpart, the neurological structure that is the brain*, an integration which neuropsychoanalysis, having more to go on, effectively illustrates. It was the "unusual built-in control" of the study coupled with the investigation's longitudinal design that shed light on the complexities of development *in which "biological activities" yield dominance to "psychological meanings."* It was the unique prospective design of the study, in other words, that fostered understanding of "the interplay between environment and inherent equipment," an interchange that integrates "the pull forward, disharmonies in emerging faculties, and engagement in the overall progression"[44] to define the maturational process, by which is meant not only psychological growth and development, but the very meaning of the mental and, thereby, of subjectivity itself.[45]

The findings of the twin study "underscore the inextricable interaction between nature and nurture." Indeed, they emphasize the uselessness of the nature-nurture dichotomy by stressing the "reciprocal relationship between constitution and the environment," with each revealing aspects and dimensions of the other. Separating them only as "a heuristic device," the team notes that "Constitutional and environmental factors impact upon one another from birth on so closely and so intimately that it is often difficult to distinguish them." Thus, we read (to offer once again what was cited earlier, but is presented in its fuller context here):

> In humans, the sequence of development of the mind takes infants from a world founded in biology to one constructed from meanings. […] Development occurs in a sequence of <u>phase-dominated plateaus</u>, each hierarchically ordered. The <u>pattern or style</u> of phase emergence is determined by components of the inherent maturationally-determined program – a program, we were to discover, that reflected such strong intra-twin concordance that we came to attribute it to the genetic pool. The program introduces potential <u>new</u> ways of being, thinking and acting, a potential that is actualized by way of interactions with specific (and variable) nutrients in the surround. The interaction results in <u>experiences</u>, which become nodal points for newly evolving structures.
>
> […]
>
> Each phase ushers in novelties, new ways of thinking, feeling, being, representing and organizing stimuli into fresh meanings, and hence, not surprisingly, phases usually arise in <u>crises</u>, i.e., along with evidence of transient disequilibrations of pre-existing modes. Each newly evolving organization is influenced by antecedent phases as well as by ongoing experiences and theoretically each is more-or-less <u>time-bound</u>, i.e., what is programmed to happen must be actualized within a biologically-influenced period if there is to be an optimal outcome.

So, too, Solms, in consideration of the "objective 'solid' images of the relevant neural processes" and the "subjective feeling states that correlate with them,"[46] in consideration of the affective modality of consciousness (the biologically positive and negative valences associated with consciousness), is focused on meaning as derived from contextualization: "Consciousness samples constellations of [perceptual/cognitive] representations in order to bestow meaning on them."[47] Why? To stabilize an otherwise unstable world, to find certainty where uncertainty and potential crisis reigns, as we shall see in Chapter Two. Art (visual, literary, or other), like dreams and fantasies, is a form of testing: It is a virtual exploration of reality that allows for inference. It shares with other manifest forms of existential trial and error the push-pull of attraction and repulsion, the cathecting and decathecting associated with wish and avoidance that are evidence of the endogenous origin of curiosity, of the interrelation between how and why we know what we know, and the imaginary. And it allows for learning, a learning in accordance with the affects and associations it induces within us. I near conclusion of this chapter with Solms' statement that "Consciousness registers the state of the subject within a biological scale of values" for, like the conclusions drawn by the authors of the manuscript regarding the "pull forward," it integrates the mind-brain duality and carries us onward.[48]

Had it been published, the manuscript on child development drafted by Neubauer, Abrams, and Balzert would seemingly have gone a long way toward deconstructing the dichotomy of the biological vs. the environmental, which is to say the nature-nurture schism with which many (knowingly or not) continue to grapple today. Even more remarkable, perhaps, is that what the manuscript shares with the recent neuropsychoanalytic writings of Solms and others is, in a word, what Sartre famously proclaimed in his 1946 defense of existentialism against its critics of the time: "Existence precedes essence."[49] No more than Solms was he proclaiming the human infant "a blank slate," but that the moral imperative to be aware of one's fundamental freedom, to accept responsibility for one's choices and actions, is the product of self-awareness, of feeling, of the subjectivity that is within us from the start. If, for the neuropsychoanalyst, "we are born with a set of innate needs" and "the main task of mental development is to learn how to meet our needs in the world," if we do so by predicting what will allow us to meet our needs and by learning from our prediction errors, it is that the "sentient subject is first and foremost an *affective* subject." Only by *feeling* our needs, by subjectively experiencing them, can we represent them consciously. Moreover, as Solms makes eminently clear, we have "*indirect* ways of meeting our needs. This often involves *substitute-formation*. Humans have a large capacity [...] for temporarily satisfying their needs in *imaginary* and *symbolic* ways."[50] Similarly, taking the proclamation "Existence precedes essence" one step beyond the moral imposed on individuals by the fundamental freedom implied therein, one step further toward the notion that to speak is to act ("parler, c'est agir" which became with Simone de Beauvoir "Écrire, c'est agir"), we arrive with Sartre, as with the neuropsychoanalyst, at the valorization of imagination itself.

Notes

1 Cited by Jonathan Cott in "Susan Sontag: The Rolling Stone Interview" (October 4, 1979), https://www.rollingstone.com/culture/culture-news/susan-sontag-the-rolling-stone-interview-41717/4/
2 As this is an unpublished draft, no page numbers will be cited.
3 Asijit Datta and Jonathan Boulter, "Samuel Beckett and Posthuman Spaces," *Textual Practice* (January 16, 2025): 10. DOI: 10.1080/0950236X.2025.2453645
4 Paul Davies, *The Demon in the Machine: How Hidden Webs of Information Are Solving the Mystery of Life* (Allen Lane, 2019), 184. Cited by Mark Solms, *The Hidden Spring: A Journey to the Source of Consciousness* (W.W. Norton, 2021), 238.
5 David Chalmers, "Facing Up to the Problem of Consciousness," *Journal of Consciousness Studies* 2, no. 3 (1995): 200–219.
6 Chalmers, "Facing Up to the Problem of Consciousness," 201.
7 Chalmers, "Facing Up to the Problem of Consciousness," 201.
8 Solms, *The Hidden Spring*, 241.
9 See Samuel Abrams, "Disposition and the Environment," *The Psychoanalytic Study of the Child* 41, no. 1 (1986): 41–60; Peter Neubauer and Alexander Neubauer, *Nature's Thumbprint: The New Genetics of Personality* (Columbia University Press, 1990); Samuel Abrams and Peter Neubauer, "Hartmann's Vision: Identical Twins and Developmental Organizations," *The Psychoanalytic Study of the Child* 49 (1994): 49–59; Peter Neubauer and Christa Balzert, *Der psychoanalytische Prozeß*, ed. Sylvia Zwettler-Otte and Albrecht Komarek (Turia + Kant, 1994). All four publications were drawn from results of the study. In addition, several presentations devoted to the study outcomes have taken place. To cite but two (both from 2003), Christa Balzert, "Genetic Findings and Their Impact on the Psychoanalytic Theory of Development," presented at the Institute for Child, Adolescent and Family Studies in New York, and Peter Neubauer and Christa Balzert, "Genetics and Psychotherapy," presented at a meeting of The American Academy of Psychoanalysis.
10 When certain of the subjects became known to each other as young adults, the media came down hard on the ethical questions associated with the separation of the children (often misrepresenting the facts and unjustifiably accusing Neubauer, whatever one's position on the issues involved). Two films (purporting to be documentaries), television, and the press all played into the spectacular nature of the similarities the twins and one set of triplets exhibited as adults having been raised apart. Yet what might well have been at the forefront of all the attention was not: It is not what those similarities *look like* that matters, but *what they mean*. And this is precisely what is spelled out in the manuscript in question, a draft left unpublished for being too revelatory of the individual subjects, a reason one can only respect.
11 See Leon Hoffman and Lois Oppenheim, "Three Identical Strangers and The Twinning Reaction: Clarifying History and Lessons for Today from Peter Neubauer's Twins Study," *JAMA* 322, no. 1 (2019): 10–12.
12 "Becoming Mind: Identical Twins Reared Apart." All subsequent unreferenced citations are from this manuscript. I am exceedingly grateful to Christa Balzert for permission to publish all quotations from the unpublished manuscript.

13 Balzert, "Genetic Findings and Their Impact on the Psychoanalytic Theory of Development," n.p.
14 Balzert, "Genetic Findings and Their Impact on the Psychoanalytic Theory of Development," n.p.
15 Abrams, "Disposition and the Environment," 55–56.
16 Emphasis added.
17 See, for example, Mark Solms, "Consciousness by Surprise: A Neuropsychoanalytic Approach to the Hard Problem," in Biophysics of Consciousness: A Foundational Approach, ed. Roman Poznanski, Jack Tuszynski, and Todd E. Feinberg (World Scientific, 2016), 129–48. https://doi.org/10.1142/9789814644266_0004 . Also, Solms, *The Hidden Spring*, especially 265–66.
18 Mark Solms and Margaret R. Zellner, "Freudian Affect Theory Today," in *From the Couch to the Lab: Trends in Psychodynamic Neuroscience*, ed. Aikaterini Fotopoulou, Donald Pfaff, and Martin Conway (Oxford University Press, 2012), 134–35.
19 Solms and Zellner, "Freudian Affect Theory Today," 135.
20 Jaak Panksepp and Lucy Biven, "A Meditation on the Affective Neuroscientific View of Human and Animalian MindBrains," in *From the Couch to the Lab: Trends in Psychodynamic Neuroscience*, 148.
21 See Mark Solms and Oliver Turnbull, "What is Neuropsychoanalysis?" *Neuropsychoanalysis* 13, no. 2 (2011): 136.
22 Solms, "Consciousness by Surprise: A Neuropsychoanalytic Approach to the Hard Problem."
23 Mark Solms, "New Project for a Scientific Psychology: General Scheme," *Neuropsychoanalysis* 22, no. 1–2 (2020): 6.
24 Solms, "New Project for a Scientific Psychology," 5.
25 As Solms has put it, "the primary *experience* of our existence is registered as affect, before we *reflect* on it." "Perspectives on Consciousness Lionel Naccache and Mark Solms," NPSA-association-org. Neuropsychoanalysis around the World Again (2021). See Chapter 2 for further elaboration of this concept.
26 Ross M. Skelton, ed., *The Edinburgh International Encyclopaedia of Psychoanalysis* (Edinburgh University Press, 2006).
27 Sigmund Freud, "A Note on the Unconscious in Psycho-Analysis," *Standard Edition*, vol. 12, 263.
28 Lois Oppenheim, "The Lexicographer's Nightmare," in *From the Couch to the Lab: Trends in Psychodynamic Neuroscience*, 282–92.
29 Edmund Husserl, *Phenomenology and the Crisis of Philosophy*, trans. Quentin Lauer (Harper & Row, 1935/1965), 190, n. 58.
30 Paul Ricoeur, *Freud and Philosophy: An Essay on Interpretation*, trans. Denis Savage (New Haven: Yale University Press, 1970), 379, 378.
31 Vittorio Gallese, "Bodily Self and Interpersonal Relations in Schizophrenia," webinar of The Neuropsychoanalysis Association, January 20, 2023.
32 Mark Solms, "Empathy as Developmental Achievement: Beyond Embodied Simulation," *Neuroscience and Critique*, ed. Jan De Vos and Ed Pluth (Routledge, 2016), 207, 204.
33 Thomas Nagel, "What Is It Like To Be a Bat?" *The Philosophical Review* 83, no. 4 (1974): 436.
34 See, for example, Solms, *The Hidden Spring*, 261.
35 Nagel, "What Is It Like To Be a Bat?," 449.
36 James Joyce, *Ulysses* (Shakespeare and Company, 1922), 3.366–67.
37 See Solms, *The Hidden Spring*, 250.
38 Thomas Szanto and Hilge Landweer, eds., *The Routledge Handbook of Phenomenology of Emotion* (Routledge, 2011), 9.

39 See, for example, Mark Solms and Oliver Turnbull, *The Brain and the Inner World* (Other Press, 2002), and Antonio Damasio, *The Strange Order of Things: Life, Feeling, and the Making of Cultures* (Pantheon, 2018).
40 Personal communication.
41 Thomas Ogden, "Rethinking the Concepts of the Unconscious and Analytic Time," *JAPA* 69, no. 1 (2021): 222.
42 Bruno Clément, *Henri Bergson, Prix Nobel de littérature* (Verdier, 2021), 40.
43 Abrams, "Disposition and the Environment," 56–57.
44 Christa Balzert, cited by Lois Oppenheim, "Review of Neubauer Twin Study: An Interview about a Controversy or a Controversial Interview?" *International Journal of Controversial Discussions* 1 (2020), 183. A small portion of the opening of this chapter may be found in that earlier text. I thank that journal editor for permission to reprint it here.
45 Once again, I take no position on any of the ethical questions that have been raised with regard to the study. Those in no way whatsoever relate to my interest in the findings as expressed in the manuscript discussed here.
46 Solms, "Consciousness by Surprise."
47 Mark Solms, "A Neuropsychoanalytic Approach to the Hard Problem of Consciousness," 10. Electronic version of article published as *Journal of Integrative Neuroscience* 13, no. 2 (2014): 173–85. DOI: doi:10.1142/S0219635214400032
48 Solms, "A Neuropsychoanalytic Approach to the Hard Problem of Consciousness."
49 Jean-Paul Sartre, *L'Existentialisme est un humanisme* (Les Éditions Nagel, 1946), 21 (trans. mine).
50 Mark Solms, "The Neurobiological Underpinnings of Psychoanalytic Theory and Therapy," *Frontiers in Behavioral Neuroscience* 12 (2018): article 294. DOI: 10.3389/fnbeh.2018.00294

Chapter 2

Beyond "Beyond the Pleasure Principle"

In their unpublished manuscript, Neubauer, Abrams, and Balzert underscore the progression of the mind, the "pull forward" that accounts for development, which is to say maturation of the individual and the sense of self. Focusing on the components that allow for the growth of the mind – on "the continuities, the discontinuities, and the functions of assembly," on "the actualization of the potential provided by what is inherent," on the genetic and congenital origins of disposition and their epigenetic variables, on the development of agency – they address the constitutional needs facilitated (as well as remedied) by the environment. They lend observational weight to what Damasio would call the "emergence of mind, feeling, and consciousness"[1] from the bidirectional interaction between the brain and body. They lend observational weight, in a word, to Frank Sulloway's description of Freud as a "biologist of the mind."[2] They predicate their understanding of the maturation of the mind, moreover, on the development of meaning, for how we contextualize experience, how we frame and, above all, learn from it, is how meaning is continually rendered, allowing for the individual *to continually become* who they are.

It is important to recognize with the authors of that manuscript the notion of *becoming*, for, in anticipation of much contemporary interdisciplinary neuroscience, it is in conceiving of development in terms of the emergence of mental function within a biological context that development is distinguished from a predominantly deterministic point of view (whether nature or nurture) and shown to account for the continuities and discontinuities that are the basis of maturation. Moreover, and even more to the point, one never *is* who one is; one evolves by necessity in accordance with the feelings, needs, and energic forces that keep us alive. As François Ansermet and Pierre Magistretti have written, "The term *becoming* enables us to show the fortuitous nature of the result of a mental evolution. What we have to do is explain what occurred in order for a new state to be constituted by starting from a line of thinking that connects continuity and discontinuity. We may be saturated with determinants, but the connection between these determinants is not entirely determined."[3]

DOI: 10.4324/9781003566755-3

Neubauer, Abrams, and Balzert's understanding of psychic evolution anticipates the notion of the mind as what Solms calls the very "being of the body."[4] As though in response to Solms' questioning of what it is that "sentient subjectivity" (as he would come to refer to it) does and how it emerges, without deterministically reducing development to psychology or psychology to physiology and in recognition of the mind and brain as inherently one, the authors offer a stunning depiction of how the "pull forward" performs in the service of biology. They offer a stunning depiction of the actual meaning of drive as a motivational force distinct from the more automatous reaction that is instinct (a distinction brought to light by Solms' retranslation of the German *trieb* in the *Revised Standard Edition* of Freud's work).

Ultimately, it would be Solms' revision of Freud's metapsychology as a "meta*neuro*psychology," the valuation of Freud's work enriched by the modernization of scientific tools for the understanding of brain function, that would provide further evidence that, as Solms puts it, "The *activated* brain is the same thing as the *feeling* mind."[5] Arrived at via observational study or the methods of neuroscience, it is the understanding of brain activation in view of the feeling mind and an understanding of both as residing in the energic force, the motivated urge referred to as drive, that is the primary conclusion of each approach. But two questions come to the fore: What *is* this "pull forward" that literally drives development? What, in other words, constitutes this "inherent impetus" (Abrams' term) that is dispositionally oriented but environmentally acted upon and that is primordially linked to consciousness and thereby to affect? And what has it to do with the interrelation between curiosity, creativity, and their less evident, but by no means less significant, counterpart, crisis? Exploring these questions will allow for an appreciation of *how determinism* (scientific, philosophical, and aesthetic alike) – the theoretical antithesis of which constitutes the core of this book – is negated by *the advent of modernism*.

The Homeostatic Function of Drive

"[E]at or be eaten!" is how the physiologist H.W. Smith explained survival.[6] The reality according to which mammals survive is homeostasis, the process of maintaining the neurochemical equilibrium, the internal balance, that, by way of feeling, keeps us alive. In his 1915 paper "Instincts and Their Vicissitudes," Freud differentiated between the so-called ego (self-preservative) and sexual (object-related) instincts. Some five years later, in "Beyond the Pleasure Principle," distinguishing between the "ego instincts" destructively oriented toward the inorganic state preceding life and thereby non-life or death and the "sexual instincts" narcissistically oriented toward the furtherance of life, he redefined the opposition, acknowledging the hypothetical status of his description and citing the insufficiency of our knowledge of biology at the time of his writing. Consistent throughout, however, were the energic processes somatic in origin and pleasure driven, pleasure understood as a lessening (or at least constancy) of the level of excitation (of "the demand made upon the mind for work in consequence of its connection with the body") and unpleasure as its quantitative increase.[7] Therein resided, according to Freud, the developmental motivation, the advancement from one phase of maturation to the next.

As is well known, Freudian drive theory, strongly contested at the time of its inception, remains controversial today. Solms, however, while posing questions to which the Neubauer, Abrams, and Balzert unpublished manuscript uncannily appears to respond, and while closely allying himself with the Freudian perspective that was clearly theirs, has revised much of Freud's early work and done so in ways of which the authors of the manuscript, as well as Freud himself, would, one has every reason to believe, strongly approve. Solms' evocation of a statement by Oliver Sacks is confirmational in this regard: "Neuropsychology, like classical neurology, aims to be entirely objective, and its great power, its advances, come from just this. But a living creature, and especially a human being, is first and last active – a subject, not an object. It is precisely the subject, the living 'I,' which is being excluded. Neuropsychology is admirable," Sacks concluded, "but it excludes the psyche – it excludes the experiencing, active, living 'I'."[8] The life of the mind is lived,[9] Solms reminds us in agreement with Sacks' observation, and it is precisely in recognition of this not-so-obvious-yet-utterly-blatant actuality that neuropsychoanalysis, incorporating psychoanalytic insight as well as neuroscientific data, came to be. And, indeed, Freud, whose early research was in neurology and neuroanatomy and in neuroscience more generally, whence the development of his psychology, predicted as much: "we must recollect that all our provisional ideas in psychology will presumably some day be based on an organic substructure."[10]

Solms has offered that substructure situating, in opposition to the corticocentric notion of consciousness, Freud's "system 'unconscious' in the non-declarative memory systems located beneath the cortex, primarily in the basal ganglia, and cerebellum."[11] He has offered that substructure determining the id "intrinsically conscious."[12] And he has offered that substructure by updating several of Freud's theoretical premises: In "New Project for a Scientific Psychology: General Scheme," for instance, "free energy" replaces the concept of "quantity," "prediction error" is substituted for "sensory excitation," and so on, while in "Revision of Drive Theory," in addition to distinguishing between "emotional" and "bodily" drives, and offering evidence of the drives as conscious, he offers reason to eliminate the death drive, and more.

Perhaps the most fundamental revision, however, concerns the pleasure principle, Solms' taking us beyond the "beyond" to which Freud referred when he conceived of the drive toward quiescence, the death instinct otherwise known as the Nirvana principle. Freud's idea that there are inclinations more primitive than the pleasure principle – that are beyond it in the sense that, as he put it, there are "tendencies more primitive than it and independent of it," tendencies the consequence of which are not always pleasurable[13] – is significantly modified by Solms' view of the many kinds of pleasure that exist in addition to those that are libidinal. Illustrating in a variety of contexts that Freud's pleasure principle falls short in not recognizing that pleasure resides in the context of non-sexual as well as sexual drives, Solms argues that the primary maturational task involves not a progression from one to the other (as in Freud's oral, anal, and phallic stages of development), but the capacity to meet our instinctual bodily and emotional needs and to integrate them whether pleasure-oriented or not. Whereas the pleasure principle for Freud derived from the maintenance of a low level of excitation, with the "beyond" emanating from more primitive, destructive instincts unrelated to that pleasure, for Solms, who goes beyond Freud's "beyond," it is a matter of learning how to reconcile the drives with each other. Whereas Freud, in other words, viewed drive more simply as regulating, Solms equates it from the start with feeling: It is drive, he maintains, that "literally brings the mind into being."[14] And it is this that accounts for "becoming," as considered by Neubauer, Abrams, and Balzert; becoming as distinct from emergence in the ordinary sense of the word. The philosopher Gilbert Simondon spoke of "becoming" in an ontologically comparable way: "In a theory of the phases of being, becoming is something other than an alteration or a succession of states comparable to a serial development. Becoming is in effect a perpetuated and renovated resolution, an incorporating resolution, proceeding through crises, such that its sense is in its center, not at its origin or its end."[15]

It is not my purpose, however, to review Solms' substantial modifications in detail here. Nevertheless, two points in particular, each made by Solms in his "Revision of Drive Theory" and incorporating the revisions of Freud's "Project" (as that work has become known), take us directly from the "becoming" of mind, the empirical progression toward relative equilibrium ("relative" insofar as resistance to the destabilizing force of uncertainty, of entropy or unpredictability, is perpetual, not transitory), to the crux of the interrelation in question. *These two points, moreover, by taking us to the core of the interconnection between curiosity, creativity, and crisis, will put in high relief the "pull forward" or "inherent impetus" that is not only maturational but the life force itself.*

The first concerns what might be considered the perfunctory role of drives. At what Solms terms a "mechanistic level," drives are both homeostatic and anti-entropic (or tending toward certainty and order).[16] Based on the empirical notion of lived experience from which learning derives, the homeostatic or "preservative" function is supported by the notion of prediction: "We do not learn just because we can," Solms tells us, "but because we must. We learn how to meet our needs in the world." And taken to the next step, this homeostatic function reveals the value of memories whose content is the past, but whose reason for being is the future: prediction, based upon the past, of what is to come.[17] Learning is not for the sake of learning, but for the purpose of establishing "optimal predictions," predictions that serve us by informing us how best to "meet our needs in a given environment." We need to learn to reconcile our predictions with what we experience. Because innate predictions may be at variance with one another, learning is required to achieve compromise between, for example, curiosity and fear or attachment and rage, as Solms has suggested. The very work of *becoming*, what Solms calls the "great task of mental development," is the supplementing of "instinctual predictions about how these multiple drive demands may be satisfied *and reconciled with each other* in unpredicted contexts."[18] And this is where imagination (among other capacities increased by learning, such as substitute-formation and the delay of gratification) comes to the fore.[19]

Referencing Friston's Free Energy Principle – the theory (highly complex and grossly over-simplified here) that our innate tendency to disorder (entropy) is reduced by the accuracy of sensorial prediction and the consequent minimization of surprise – Solms locates the homeostatic function of drive. In the paradigm offered by Friston, he situates the life-preserving motivation for the psychic "pull forward" recognized observationally as such by Neubauer, Abrams, and Balzert. Friston's theory stems from the second law of thermodynamics which states that in any closed system the degree of entropy, or disorder and dissolution, increases or remains constant. And all living entities aggressively oppose it. Friston accounts for this opposition in what he describes as a drive to reduce the disconnect between sensory input and expectation, in the minimization of free energy.

Stemming from the hypothesis proposed by the eighteenth-century English statistician and clergyman Thomas Bayes – a hypothesis known as "the Bayes theorem" which reveals how the brain, in continuous struggle against surprise for the purpose of maintaining homeostatic equilibrium, prevails – Friston's Free Energy Principle is increasingly the premise upon which neuroscience (with psychiatry not far behind) is based. And, more recently, applying Friston's innovations in brain imaging and his understanding of abnormalities in both structural and functional cerebral activity, Friston and Solms have begun applying Bayes' probability theory, its relevance to the psyche's furtherance of the biological, to Artificial Intelligence. At the root of these endeavors, in short, is the idea that it is by tracing aspects of the world – and constructing thereby a model that allows for its navigation in such a way as to reduce any incongruity between the actuality of experience and the predictions emanating from that model – that we minimize errors of expectation. This is to say that the source of the "pull forward" is the prototype created from sensory input along with anticipation relating to the prototype, errors relating to anticipation, and corrections to guarantee its realization. To cite Friston himself, the Free Energy Principle is the idea "that any (biological) system that conserves its form must minimize 'surprise'," which is to say "maximize adaptive fitness" by way of "exchange with its environment."[20] Briefly put, the principle formulates the tendency to disorder inherent in all "biological agents, like animals or brains"[21] and the homeostatic need for its resistance. The minimization of uncertainty, the direct result of prediction, is precisely in the service of this homeostatic need. *The minimization of uncertainty is thus the shield against the turning point to which prediction error leads, the very shield against crisis itself.*

The second point concerns the governing role of affect. While Freud appreciated that the demands referred to as drives are ultimately experienced affectively, what he did not recognize, according to Solms, "is that such demands are actually felt at their *source.*" Affect, in other words, is "the *subjective* aspect of 'drive.'"[22] In agreement with neuroscientist Jaak Panksepp who defined, in addition to bodily drives, the seven emotional drive systems referred to briefly in the preceding chapter – SEEKING, RAGE, FEAR, LUST, CARE, PANIC/GRIEF, PLAY (capitalized as in Panksepp's own writings to set them apart from their colloquial usage[23]) – Solms emphasizes the association of all drives with affect illustrating the origin of their conscious representation (as opposed to conceptualization) and their homeostatic reason for being. This is to say that, like Panksepp, Solms views drives as both *felt* and *consciously represented* in the service of their fundamental objective: defending against destabilization through the minimization of free energy, through the resistance that optimizes prediction accuracy. Homeostatic and linked with affect, drives, in sum, are the tools with which we combat uncertainty, with which we diminish surprise.

Why such agents minimize free energy by altering their expectations, by reducing the element of surprise is, in other words, explained by feeling: Unlike those in neuroscience who claim that a concept of a given feeling must precede the experience of that feeling, those who subscribe to what Lisa Feldman Barrett calls "the theory of constructed emotion," a theory based on the coming together of social, psychological, and neuro constructions to create categories of emotional response that are learned, Solms and Panksepp, among others, speak to the *innate origin of affect.* Rather than constructing categories of affective states by way of conceptual knowledge about emotion, they view emotion, which implicates a conscious awareness of it, as instinctively stemming from sensory input, from the responsiveness of brain circuits to experiential triggers.[24] And it is in conjunction with Panksepp's basic emotional systems and Friston's principle of free energy that Solms revised Freud's drive theory and updated the "Project" as well. But it is where all this takes us that will allow me to advance the primary argument I wish to put forth, an argument having to do with *the misconstruing on the aesthetic front the consequences of revising Freud, the misconstruing on the aesthetic front the consequences of conceiving of a metaneuropsychology in view of Panksepp's idea of drive and Friston's predictive coding.*

From Homeostatic Need to Aesthetic Pleasure

I spoke at the start of this book of the "krisis" identified by Husserl, the crisis of Western culture – or, more precisely, of the European sciences – abusive of the subjectivity of humankind. I spoke of the existential crisis identified by Sartre and later by Kristeva, among others, as a crisis of inattention: a lack of awareness on the part of the individual of their fundamental freedom, their freedom to choose, to act, to imagine and thereby to create and to revolt as well. And I have now spoken of the crisis related to the failure to effectively minimize the errors of prediction by which we lead our lives, crisis being endemic to the endogenous, fundamentally affective, and self-organizing objective of self-preservation. I have briefly spoken, in other words, of the crisis that threatens our equilibrium when the neuronal encoding of expectation relating to sensory input is not continually updated, when uncertainty is not minimized and prediction error not continually revised, "continually" being the operative word in the very sense of the "becoming of mind." But what protects us against all three – the crisis of scientific positivism (at the expense of consciousness), the crisis of inattention (to freedom and responsibility), and the crisis of uncertainty (of entropic minimization) – is curiosity. *What protects us against all three is the learning – secondary to the innate nature of feeling – to which curiosity gives rise, the "pull forward" which defines the drive that is curiosity, the becoming of mind through the creativity that curiosity impels.*

Neurobiology, neurophysiology – neuroscience more generally – owe nothing to Sigmund Freud. Or so the more cognitively oriented neuroscientist would claim (although perhaps less so today than yesterday). The neural underpinnings of perceptual experience are explored by the affectively oriented neuroscientist, however, in view of the recognition that sense perception, perceptual experience, attains its degree of pleasure (hedonic valence) by virtue of emotion. It is emotion that valorizes the corporeal apprehension (visual, auditory, somatosensory).[25] It is emotion that contextualizes what has always been among humankind's greatest pleasures: aesthetic experience. As we know from Solms, it is from the relation of perception to affect that the subjectivity of conscious awareness derives. And it is in this arena that much is indeed owed Freud, for, regardless of the multiplicity of ensuing directions psychoanalysis as a treatment modality would ultimately follow, it was his theory of mind in its fundamental relation to the human body, his notion of the inherency of emotional need, of the learning obtained by way of experience and its unconscious processing, his notion of drive that would account for Solms' revision of metapsychology as a metaneuropsychology and the founding of neuropsychoanalysis. It was his notion of drive that is confirmed by Neubauer, Abrams, and Balzert's prospective (as opposed to retrospective) observational study of the "becoming" of mind, the emergence owing solely not to nature or nurture, but to the mediation of the body's set points of homeostasis as described by Panksepp and Solms. Freud inferred the existence, nature, and number of our felt drives from clinical psychological observations, but affective neuroscience has modified and corrected his inferences about them, using the additional data that is provided by physiological observations, enabled by newer research methods." (See Solms, "Revision of Drive Theory," 2021).

As mentioned previously, neuroaesthetics initially gained prominence by research, in the 1990s and early 2000s, into the visual workings of the brain. Whether having to do with the creation of the artwork or its viewing, it was the ocular circuitry and neural anatomy of the brain that informed understanding of the making and reception of visual art. In a 2011 publication, Tomohiro Ishizu and Semir Zeki moved beyond consideration of the purely visual components to distinguishing between art and beauty. Aiming to locate conceptualized style and projected truth in an arena other than that of the beautiful (and citing paintings by Francis Bacon and Lucian Freud in this regard), Ishizu and Zeki proposed aesthetic experience not only in terms of the activation of particular brain regions, but a subjective (which is to say, determined by a single individual in a particular moment and place) and quantifiable (the magnitude of activation) definition of aesthetic experience.[26] Expanding their "brain-based theory of beauty" (as they called it) toward a broader explanation of aesthetics, Ishizu and Zeki raised the question of the connection between, on the one hand, activity in the specific region of the brain (the medial orbitofrontal cortex) on which their study was focused and, on the other, reward. Noting "that activity in mOFC correlates with the experience of pleasure and reward, whether real or imagined, and its expectation," they brought to a neurobiological level "an issue *long discussed in the humanities*, namely the relationship of aesthetic experience to pleasure."[27]

Two years following this publication, which deepened and broadened the growing neuroscientific interest in the art-brain correlation, a study appeared offering a radically different explanation of the origin in which the pleasure of aesthetic experience was said to reside. No longer emphasizing the convergence between "the cortical organization of the visual nervous system and the visual attributes that artists use to express their art," the authors of this publication, Vittorio Gallese among them, claimed that "perception and action are not separate domains implemented in different anatomical and functional circuits," that perception does not precede action, but that "action itself contributes to perception." Although adhering to the principal notion of neuroaesthetics that "the activation of the visual cortex of the beholder is a crucial aspect of visual art perception," they articulated their belief in the irreducibility of the aesthetically experienced visual image either to "a cortical visual process [or] to high order cognitive processes." And in accordance with the results of a study investigating cortical motor responses to paintings by the Abstract Expressionist Franz Kline, paintings not only highly abstract, but deemed utterly "static," they made the case for cortical motor system activation during observation. The conclusion reached, in other words, supported the notion of sensorimotor arousal stimulated by the viewing of such art. It supported, as articulated by the authors, "the hypothesis postulating the role of embodied simulation of artist's gestures in the perception of his/her works of art, grounded on the activation of the physiological mirror mechanism instantiated by cortical premotor areas."[28]

Embodiment, understood in accordance with the neuronal processes both of perception and action, and embodied simulation, conceived in accordance with the arousal of such processes as a response, at once both reflective and empathic, to the emotional and corporeal sensations of another, are said to contribute to our responses to art. Such an understanding of visual artworks, attributed in large part to Gallese, has achieved considerable recognition for its extension of the cognitive perspective into the domain of the intersubjective, motor and emotional, its attributing to bodily sensation the encounter of the viewer or reader with the visual or literary work or art. Locating in various mirroring or reflective responses in the brain the activity elicited by the perception of the artist's creative process, embodied simulation accounts for the viewer's resonance with the artwork and the pleasure that results. Whether by way of memory or association, the observer, like the artist with whom an intersubjective exchange is said to be initiated, is, in a sense, a co-creator of the work. In the context of embodied simulation, the mind, itself embodied, partakes not only of an intersubjective but an intercorporeal exchange.[29] Crediting the fundamental connection between the beholder and artist to empathic activation of the sensorimotor system, to the arousal of emotional and motor processes to which the neuronal circuitry gives rise, aesthetic experience as seen from this perspective responds to the so-called "hard problem" of the brain-to-mind correlation.

Contrary to Gallese, however, Solms, for one, attributes embodied simulation to mechanisms considerably more reflective than compassionate, the former occurring automatically via mirror neurons, the latter acquired as opposed to innate and best considered a feat of development. While not denying the existence of embodied simulation, Solms situates this "mirroring mechanism" on another level of function, one not truly empathic in the accurate (if complex) sense of the term and outside the aesthetic domain. "Artworks are actually as dead as doornails," Solms proclaims. "It is possible to misperceive the state of another mind in ways that do not arise with, say, the appreciation of a landscape. Who is to say whether or not a willow is weeping?"[30] But I will return to this later. For the moment, suffice it to say that – while there are paintings and there is performance art, while there is music and there is literature, and the idea of empathy as it relates to aesthetics may vary accordingly – aesthetic pleasure may be said to emanate from engagement (reflective, empathic, or some combination thereof) by way of the energic force that is drive.

Two Emotional Drive Systems

Writing of children's play in "Beyond the Pleasure Principle," Freud describes the pleasure to be found in pretending:

> It is clear that in their play children repeat everything that has made a great impression on them in real life, and that in doing so they abreact the strength of the impression and, as one might put it, make themselves master of the situation. [...] It can also be observed that the unpleasurable nature of an experience does not always unsuit it for play. If the doctor looks down a child's throat or carries out some small operation on him, we may be quite sure that these frightening experiences will be the subject of the next game; but we must not in that connection overlook the fact that there is a yield of pleasure from another source. As the child passes over from the passivity of the experience to the activity of the game, he hands on the disagreeable experience to one of his playmates and in this way revenges himself on a substitute.[31]

And, likening artistic imitation to the pretend of child's play, he offers what he considers to be proof of the dominance of the need for pleasure (the enjoyment of the audience before the theatrical performance, for example, even of a tragedy) only to move past it to the more primitive tendency of which he now conceived, the death instinct (or Thanatos, as opposed to Eros, the life instinct in Freud's dual-instinct theory).

Conversely, Solms, in persuasively arguing that all drives are fundamentally homeostatic or life-preserving, demonstrates their objective as satiation, the fulfillment of need, not pleasure.[32] It was in falsely equating the two, he maintains, that Freud erroneously arrived at this drive which is utterly deconstructed by the pull of homeostasis, the energic force toward those set points that maintain equilibrium. Interestingly, it was a painter – a highly abstract painter – who would term the anti-entropic nature of this instinctual force, the homeostatic quest, the "drive of Becomingness":

> Beginning with the magical art of primitive times, man has always attempted to stem the drive of Becomingness by fixing his attention and efforts upon an emotion or an object, in order to preserve it from time and flux and change.[33]

One may or may not view art, and our forever history of making it, as an indirect result of the drive of emergence, the idea that one resists the "pull forward" in the effort to counter the movement in time toward "flux and change," toward entropy and even non-being. But the point made by John Day (1932–1982) certainly appears to exemplify the notion that art is anti-entropic. And, in his own paintings, particularly those of his later years, he reveals a deep preoccupation with the need for certainty while exposing simultaneously the freely energic drive that it opposes.

Figure 2.1 John Day, "SUMMER – 1821 –" (46 inches x 40 inches). ©John Day, 1979. (Private collection). With permission of Iain Brunt of the John Day artist estate.

In the most abstract paintings of John Day, it is constancy and variability, visibility and invisibility, color and its dematerialization, that provide both form and content.[34] The late paintings, the artist explained in comparing this work to his earlier paintings, "are still constructed and ordered, and still they are developed from contrasts of variables and constants – the play between colors, the transitions between and amongst them."[35] While harmony and purity characterize his vision, above all the abstract work of his last years, it is precisely this "play" that is of unique significance, this "play" that takes place at the intersection of light and darkness, of containment and freedom, as art critic Helen Harrison would describe Day's work.[36] "My aim is to paint paintings so quiet you can hear a pin drop," Day said of his later work, for he determined that his earlier paintings were "too busy": "They're Berlioz. I want to be Bach."[37] And indeed there is a "musical structure," as Iian Michael Brunt would say of Day's art, a geometrization that the painter's assistant, Robert Napolitano, explained as "'a family of colours based on mathematical sequences, with two parent colours (numbered 1 and 9) at the end of the scale, and a middle fifth colour created by mixing various amounts of the parent colours together in the same daylight.'"[38] Writing of a posthumous show of Day's work, Harrison also noted the absence over time of figuration, of illusion, in favor of the rhythm constituted by the modulation of tonalities, of the tensions contained within the geometrization of colored spaces.[39]

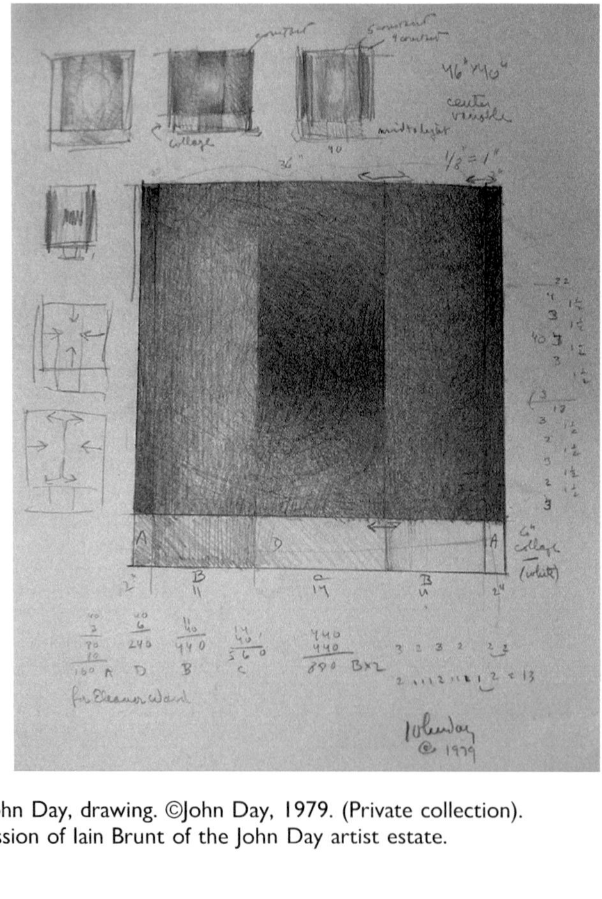

Figure 2.2 John Day, drawing. ©John Day, 1979. (Private collection). With permission of Iain Brunt of the John Day artist estate.

To David Shirey (also writing of a posthumous, though somewhat earlier, exhibit of Day's painting), the same play – a play with the equivocal, the uncertain – dominates the artist's late work. The subtlety of the imaginative usage of color and light contrasted with their rigorous organization by Day provides for a play of tonalities at once rigorous and transcendent.[40] And, in fact, the measured exactitude as related to color, contrast, size of one or another hue – all was worked out by the artist in advance.

To understand the origin of Day's computational arrangements which lend order and certainty, to understand the tensions that provide rhythmicity to the ambiguity that is disorder and uncertainty, one would not need to consider Day's work from a psychobiographical perspective (a perspective to which, as I discuss in Chapter Five, I am generally opposed), but to have the artist (as opposed to his work) on the couch. What can be said, though, is that in his particular form of creative expression there is something very evident to which the above-named critics allude, something of which the artist himself was very aware: Representing both a pleasure and a need, the teasing of the aforementioned hues, contrasts, colors, and transitions as well, all put in high relief the drive that is PLAY.

PLAY (once again, capitalized here as it was by Jaak Panksepp to differentiate it, and all other of the seven emotional brain systems he identified, from its quotidian usage) is difficult to define. It was conceived by Panksepp not as a drive as such (a notion which carries with it a sense of redundancy, for it is by definition a force; it is, in its essence, energic, which is to say driven), but as a "bodily *need state*,"[41] a motivational state affectively experienced as pleasurable, joyful, and, like all the emotional systems, not only homeostatically beneficial but essential. How, though, does child's play, for example, fulfill a physiological need? And, more to the point, how does such fulfillment relate to aesthetic experience? What, in a word, has art to do with PLAY? The answer, simply put, is to be found in the unreality and in the enactment of each. "[Reflecting] genetically ingrained ludic impulses of the nervous system,"[42] Panksepp noted, and requiring an environment devoid of fear, hunger, and other inhibitors, PLAY, like dreaming, like fantasizing, allows for a testing of reality, of engagement with others and real-life circumstances, a testing that is variable in meaning, magical, and stimulating. The neural circuits relating to PLAY, its neuroanatomy and neurochemistry as well, have been identified by those aiming to reveal the meaning of joy, of its expression in laughter, of its service to maturation, as well as its inhibition by fear and other negative emotions. But what has most recently come to the fore in the understanding of PLAY is just how much its unreality, its being imaginative, serves the purpose of diminishing uncertainty. PLAY allows for prediction based on trial and error of no *real* consequence; it allows for the apperception of probability and hence expectation, the reduction of what Friston made known in his Free Energy Principle as the minimization of entropy. And it thereby allows for the expansion of resilience, the regulation of emotion, an enhancement of agency and a resulting sense of pleasure.

We saw in the previous chapter how Solms locates affect at the core of consciousness. So, too, Panksepp has shown how seven emotional systems reveal our capacity to subjectively *feel* the interplay of our neural circuitry. And Friston has revealed the critical function of the minimization of free energy, which is to say the importance of its role in maintaining homeostasis via the reduction of uncertainty. In making the point that "consciousness" itself "is felt *uncertainty*," Solms has stated, simply and directly, that "increasing uncertainty in relation to any biological imperative *just* is 'bad' from the (first-person) perspective of such an organism [...] while decreasing uncertainty *just* is 'good.'"[43] And therein lies the relation of PLAY to the biological understanding of human mental function, to psychoneurological development, to behavior inherently creative. And thereby its relation to art as well: art shares with PLAY the primary feature of being unreal and all that implies. "Being present as an interested spectator at a spectacle or play does for adults what play does for children," Freud wrote in a posthumously published paper,[44] highlighting the magical element of illusion that play, like visual art, provides. Unlike science, art engages with the unknowable. And with surprisal as well,[45] the *unknowable* and *surprisal* being related but not one and the same.

By no means restricted to games and the like, PLAY is the first "incentive system"[46] (to cite Panksepp's preferred term) of evident relevance to the "what if," the "as if," the not real or imagined. Allowing for the origination, if not the certainty, of new predictions, pretending, as one kind of PLAY, constitutes a very significant role in child development precisely for its enhancement of the capacity to generate a range or multiplicity of new ideas. Symbolism, whether in pretend play or artistic endeavors, fosters various kinds of creative substitutes for the real and the concrete. So, too, the presymbolic (as we shall see in Chapter Four). Linguistic figures of speech, such as metaphor, are part and parcel of PLAY. As is affect: Pleasure, joy, sadness and other forms of affective engagement, including empathy, occur in PLAY. While one might not agree with the notion that the pleasure of PLAY necessarily resides in the reduction of surprise, of prediction error, as some theorists of play experience proclaim,[47] the ludic urge, with its de-stressing effects, would appear to occupy a significant place in creativity where *surprise is actually central to the pleasure involved.*

"Combinatory play," defined by psychoanalyst Victoria Stevens as "the conscious and unconscious cognitive playful manipulation of two or more ideas, feelings, sensory experiences, images, sounds, words, or objects," is a case in point. This kind of mental play has players experimenting with hypotheses, with variable conclusions, and adjusting to "unexpected results and even 'failures.'" In other kinds of creative activity as well, play involves not only "thoughtful risk taking," but the questioning of expectations and the use of errors for learning. "Creativity does not merely depend on the emotional ability to tolerate uncertainty, ambiguity, and not knowing," writes

Stevens, "but also on the ability to play with counterfactuals and to combine possibilities into alternative realities." Imagination is about the possible, not the certain. It is "the action of forming images in visual, aural, cognitive, and emotional space of 'what could be' or 'what might be.'" Imaginative play – whether with words, concepts, or images – requires flexibility, indeed the capacity, to tolerate uncertainty and ambiguity.[48]

Much has been written on creativity and on the meaning and value (the developmental, psychological, and health-inducing effects) of play, but the relation between PLAY, in Panksepp's sense of a biologically innate affective system, a system inherently pleasurable, and aesthetic experience has been insufficiently explored. This is not to say that the benefits of all aspects of play in art have been ignored. One need but think of the post-World War II playwrights associated with the Theater of the Absurd and the number of critical treatises their work has inspired to appreciate the investigation of play in literature – the humor, the "toying" with words, the monosyllabic expressions and meaningless articulations even – and its significance in the context of broader imaginative experience. But science has only relatively recently come on board with neuroaestheticians considering the conscious and unconscious playful manipulation of ideas, feelings, sensory experience of images, sounds, and more; in short, play as integral to the creative imagination.

That Samuel Beckett's favorite word was "perhaps" helped him to aestheticize play by emphasizing its ambiguity. Characters in his novels and plays are often "unnamable," as in the novel of that name or the play *Not I* (where the sole character is Mouth), or have names of only a single amorphous letter: W, for instance (a stand-in for Woman), in *Rockaby* and L (for Listener) and R (for Reader) in *Ohio Impromptu*. Locations are un-locatable ("A country road. A tree." is where *Waiting for Godot* takes place); time is atemporal; people may be anywhere (*Endgame* has two characters in trashcans; and *Play* has three in urns); and, sometimes, "Nothing happens, twice!" (as critic Vivian Mercier famously said of the two acts of *Godot*). It is not for nothing that Beckett's 1963 play *Play* is so named. It is no more for nothing, as Angela Moorjani has observed, than his explicit likening of "painterly or writerly activity to child's play: 'Now it is a game, I am going to play,' announces Malone in *Malone Dies*, as he is about to launch into another fiction, and Hamm in *Endgame* as he labors at his story, intones: 'Then babble, babble, words, like the solitary child who turns himself into children, two, three, so as to be together, and whisper together, in the dark.'"[49] It's not for nothing that what is performed in the theater is a "play" and that one "plays" an instrument, the noun originating in the Old English plega ("to exercise") and the verb from plegian ("brisk movement") being related to the Middle Dutch pleien: to "leap for joy, to rejoice."[50] No more for nothing than the choice of *Play* and *Playing* as titles for paintings by Agnes Martin (1912–2004) created in 1966 and 1994 respectively.

"In *Play* […]," as Nancy Princenthal, Martin's biographer, has written,

> the vertical rectangles, in two sizes, are painted in cool white over a neutral, light tan ground that suggests balsa wood. This white net goes to the canvas edge but falters in some places, slightly, making it seem to hover above the ground. Its vertical lines appear to be freehand and, at points of intersection with horizontal ones, what may have been occasional pauses of the brush produce very small pools of white. Gossamer and spidery, this grid is, within the parameters of Martin's mature work, surprisingly irregular – perhaps that is the playfulness of the title.[51]

And

> In *Playing*, a strong illusion of volume is created where bands of blue are bordered below with shadow-like strips of darker blue, and above with narrow strips of bright white, which [...] creates the impression of substantial horizontal louvers, their top edges here sharply illuminated.[52]

Illusion and impression: both active ingredients of play.

My point is not that such art is comparable to the frivolity of play, but that its pleasure resides in the very sensation associated with figuring the previously unfigured. Pleasure emanates not from the representation (the re-presentation) of the external, but the localization of the pre-representational. While not describable in terms of pleasure as such, though there is pleasure in the gaining of insight and in the relief from psychic pain, the spontaneity and insight of the psychoanalytic situation may be said to offer something comparable to that of the aesthetic in this regard. Of the presentation of "foreclosed affects that correspond to states of infantile distress" in the work of Louise Bourgeois, psychoanalyst Britt-Marie Schiller has written that "The analyst can present such affects by linking, through associative chains, not what has been repressed, but what has never been psychically represented or conscious." Giving shape to what was previously inaccessible, symbolizing the pre-symbolic, creating art that gives form "to emotions and fantasies that have not been conceived or represented, but registered on a primordial unconscious level,"[53] may similarly be described as equilibrating. As Panksepp hypothesized a quarter century ago, "play is a 'neuro-tonic' that can have antistress, health-promoting effects."[54] It should also be noted that aesthetic experience focused, quite literally, on ambiguity, on uncertainty, on the undefined is precisely how many visual artists – artists associated with Minimalism, Abstract Expressionism, and other modernist movements – play.

Consider, for example, the grid: In a sense, nothing in visual art is more emblematic of PLAY than this "ambivalizing," so to speak, form-creating process associated with modern art but one used by artists as far back as Ancient Egypt. Neither perspectival (perspective alluding to the accuracy of size and physical relation to the surround) nor lacking in clarity (for the delineation of its lines render the grid the purveyor of uniformity and proportion), the grids of Agnes Martin, like those of Piet Mondrian, Mark Rothko, and others, are at once materialistic and spiritual. The sense of anonymity and the sense of spacelessness are what appealed to Martin in this form and what she was after in the limitless adjacent squares she configured ad infinitum to reach an ultimate state of non-configuration. However measured the format, nothing is more silent and silencing, more disciplined and demanding (and thereby restrictive and withholding), than the grids she, for one, repeatedly executed. Emblematic and concretizing, the grid is a form that elicits ambivalence, that *is ambivalizing*, for its "indecision about its connection to matter on the one hand or spirit on the other,"[55] as critic Rosalind Krauss has remarked. Consistent and formal, silent and certain, it elicits in the viewer the pleasure evoked by elegance and beauty. Displeasure, however, is also prompted by withholding and denial, but *not* in a way that implies either a dislike of the art or a contraindication of the pleasure evoked by Panksepp's emotional system. Rather, it is more of a vexation of the kind a child may experience in a moment of pretending when the storyline does not go their way. "The grid appears in symbolist art," Krauss observes, "in the form of windows, the material presence of their panes expressed by the geometrical intervention of the window's mullions. The symbolist interest in windows clearly reaches back into the early nineteenth century and romanticism. But in the hands of the symbolist painters and poets, this image is turned in an explicitly modernist direction. For the window is experienced as simultaneously transparent and opaque." And it is that very transparency and opacity that calls for the like and dislike, the pleasure and displeasure, what Krauss calls "the ambi- or multivalence."[56]

If the grid serves as an example of aesthetic PLAY, it is that it illustrates this emotional system as fulfilling not only overt but non-overt social functions. Abstract painting, and painting with forms as obtuse as the grid, as uncertain and "ambivalizing" as the grid, stimulate innovation in the viewer much as social play stimulates creativity in children. Innovation provides a route toward knowing and the viewer – curious to detect what it is the grid is playing with – is at play with the artist in the effort to determine the what and how of the form: Is it a structured space definable as what Krauss terms "a section of an implied continuity"? Is it "an autonomous, organic whole"? Or, as in Mondrian's work, both?[57]

Rigorous in their exactitude yet enigmatic in their undefined *raison d'être*, grids play covertly with the viewer. So, too, does all non-figurative painting. It is abstract visual art, more than any other, that confronts us with the "As if" insofar as it presents the viewer with a multiplicity of possibilities. Its forms relating in some way to this, that, or the other, it is filled with surprise given that the uncertain connotation, the uncertain value even, attributed to unrecognizable shapes of a painting are variable in accordance with the context (timing, location, mood of the viewer) in which the abstraction is viewed. I will return later to how affect and ambiguity may be further related in the aesthetic domain. For the moment, the point I wish to stress is the affective incentive of the energic system that is PLAY. As Panksepp wrote, "In more than a poetic sense, energy is delight,"[58] and PLAY is a drive consistently characterized, in one way or another, by such a reward.

The other of Panksepp's "incentive systems" of evident relevance to the "what if" – to the "as if," to the not real or imagined – is the SEEKING system. As Panksepp described it, "the SEEKING system has a characteristic feeling tone – a psychic energization that is difficult to describe but is akin to that invigorated feeling of anticipation we experience when we actively seek thrills and other rewards." As "a neuroemotional system [that] *drives* and *energizes* many mental complexities that humans experience as persistent feelings of interest," it embeds curiosity, the striving to know. And it harbors creativity as well: "[I]nitially without cognitive content, it gradually helps cement the perception of causal connections in the world and thereby creates ideas."[59] It creates ideas, the images that give rise to them, and the images derived from within them. The energizing generates pleasure upon fulfillment, as is easily understood; but not to be discounted is the pleasure accompanying the quest itself, the creativity engaged in and impelled by this incentivizing system, this motivational drive. Not to be discounted is the pleasure of the search – whether a pursuit of meaning, a quest for knowledge, a seeking of beauty – not unlike appetitive stimulation, the very search that keeps all animals alive.

Panksepp's SEEKING drive is an emotional (as opposed to bodily) drive that Solms has defined, like all drives, as homeostatic and thereby anti-entropic; more precisely, an "energetic searching 'foraging' behavior, accompanied by a conscious feeling state that may be characterized as expectancy, interest, curiosity, enthusiasm, or optimism."[60] When considered in the framework of development, it is that which motivates the mind, furthers it in its perpetual state of *becoming* (for the need to reconcile the drives with each other is an ongoing task, the mind never actually just *is*), propels it toward maturation (which never actually just ends), and protects it from crisis, the threatened state of chaos and discontinuity. In the context of aesthetic experience, SEEKING may result in experimentation with form and color that stimulates emotion and activates the brain and it may do so not only through recognition, but its absence as well. Agnes Martin was dedicated to formlessness, about which more in Chapter Four. For the moment, suffice it to say that what she called "inspiration" is what she aimed to capture, particularly in her late work, in uniquely non-representational paintings where sublimity, harmony, and a kind of ecstasy reign. "Being is what demands creation of us so that we have experience of it," wrote Merleau-Ponty.[61] Exploring being, what one might call "ontological SEEKING," is what constitutes the essence of creative exploration and Martin's work projects not the autonomy of art as depiction, but the contextualization of the viewer's own field of vision. Not constitutional of absolute meaning, which would accompany the certainty of the re-presentation of something exterior to it, but constituted experientially and thereby ambiguously, which is to say as temporally fluid, dependent upon the viewer's variable experience of the moment,

Martin's abstract painting, as Eric Kandel has said of abstract painting generally, "show[s] us the world in a completely *unfamiliar* way."[62] We will return to the consequences of this unfamiliarity in Chapter Three, but a consideration, however brief, of the painting of one other whose work both reveals the artist's SEEKING and stimulates a similar wonder and curiosity in the viewer, stimulates the viewer's own creative sensibility, will illustrate the relation of this drive and the visually aesthetic experience.

Unlike the work of others whose painting is abstract in the sense of a transformation of the actual to the indeterminate, the painting of the celebrated French painter Geneviève Asse (1923–2021) may be said to reveal looking itself. As she wrote in her own notes, "Le bleu est un appel" ("Blue is a calling"), and her use of the particular tone of blue readily associated with her work was as a language of beckoning. Summoning Asse to the Brittany of her childhood, to the sea and sky of prewar France (a France she aimed to protect as a participant in the Liberation, a participation for which she was highly honored), blue was a spatializing force, an opening, a promise of depth and interiority. It was for Asse and remains for the viewer a mode of seeing and a means of searching. As the Argentinian writer Silvia Baron Supervielle has described it:

Geneviève Asse's blue is a look. It is also the quest that guides

> her choice of format and the mixing of doses from her tubes. Her brush blends the paint in the pot, as an alchemist would, and, before spreading it on the canvas, even before exposing it to the light, she instills its contents into it.[63]

As Baron Supervielle further notes, some of Asse's works have "Fenêtre" ("Window") as a title, though all her paintings could be considered as such.[64] Windows and doors, not as exits but entrances, open onto a clarity of vision not shown in the work but present nonetheless. Drawing the viewer in by the lyricism of the brush stroke as much as by the vertical white line often only quietly apparent, her paintings, neither truly abstract nor monochromatic, are invitational in much the same way as the rhythm of music or the movement of dance draw one in. While the need to know, with the reward that is the promise of knowing, accounts for arousal in the emotional system that is SEEKING, this is not to say that SEEKING is about the avoidance of uncertainty. On the contrary, it is about actively engaging with it. And as a connection to the ambiguous, aesthetic experience is an engagement with unknowing, something which science, by definition, cannot be insofar as it requires an accumulation of research-affirming certainty. Art, however, cannot be without the fervent arousal of the SEEKING system. And if Asse's art is pleasure-filled it is precisely that there is a feeling of invigoration that emanates from desire, the desire associated with curiosity, with wanting to grasp hold of the undefined, from the vastness of what she called "her blue," and learn from it.

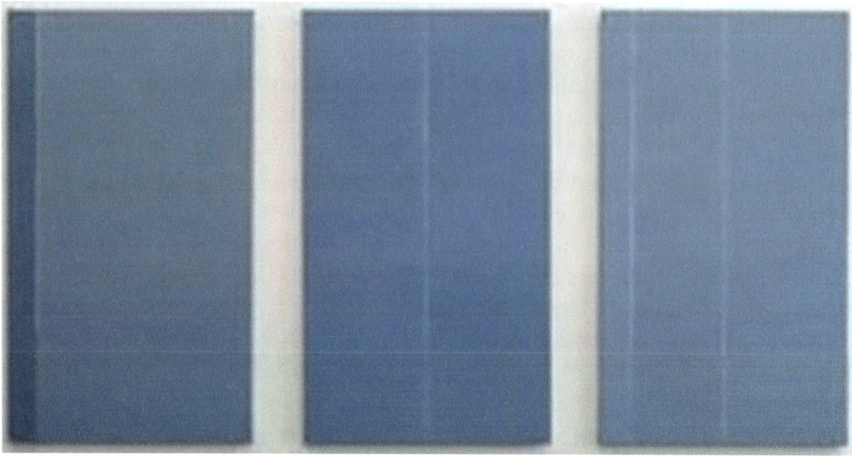

Figure 2.3 Geneviève Asse, Untitled, 1992. © 2025 Artists Rights Society (ARS), New York / ADAGP, Paris.
Courtesy of Menil Archives, The Menil Collection, Houston. Photo: Paul Hester.

Indeed, what vitalizes creativity, what discharges and ultimately assuages the tensions that maintain the SEEKING drive as a force, is the wanting, the "needing" to know. Perhaps more than any other of Panksepp's emotional systems, it is SEEKING that illustrates how, to cite Solms, "bodily needs become a mental energy."[65] Solms goes so far as to claim that "Drives are *conscious*," that they are, in fact, "the fount of all consciousness," and he notes the likeness of drive energy as defined by Freud with the variational certainty delimiting free energy as defined by Friston.[66] Indeed, Friston has, together with Robin Carhart-Harris, demonstrated the conformity of much neuroscientific theorizing (developed in conjunction with radiological imaging) with universal brain function and Freudian theory. Distinguishing between primary and secondary thought processes, describing and contrasting the neurophysiology of each – which is to say the phenomenology of the ego and the id, the former "bound," the latter "free" – Friston and Carhart-Harris attest to the validity of Freud's model and its usefulness with regard to the apprehension, in the framework of neurobiology, of clinically relevant psychological experience. In doing so, they consider essential matters deemed irreconcilable with cognitive theory. And, in proposing "that intrinsic networks self-organize into hierarchical frameworks, in order to suppress the free-energy of their subordinate levels," they expose the value to psychiatry of the substantiation of psychoanalysis by way of neuroscience.[67]

And Yet...

The emotional drive systems of the mind and the neural processes subtending them are unequivocally fundamental to artistic creation and reception.

Increasingly, they are the subject of investigation in the realm of aesthetic experience. PLAY and SEEKING, akin to any "bodily *need state*"[68] to which pleasure is homeostatically beneficial, are affectively experienced as pleasurable. Aesthetic pleasure, like the pleasure of PLAY and that of SEEKING – the one residing in the "as if" and the other in the anticipatory arousal stimulated by the quest – is generative. Like dreaming, like fantasizing, visual and literary art allow for a testing of reality, of engagement with others and real-life circumstances by being variable in sensation, stimulating, and meaningful. Visual and literary art, with the multiple types of perceptual and affective signals they generate, are integrative – enriching thereby the sense of self much as these emotional drive systems enrich development, the "pull forward" or "becoming" of mind.

"Whatever play is about," as Solms has said, "is something fundamental to what art is all about." Art, he has said, "is not real. […] it's not life. It's about life. It represents life. It evokes life. It imagines life. It reflects on life. It's a sort of 'as if' kind of life. That's what is different about art, as opposed to life. It's the lack of reality. It's the not realness about it." And yet, as Mark Rothko put it, "A painting is not a picture of an experience. It is an experience."[69] Though they might seem so at first glance, these statements are not contradictory: However "not real" a painting may be said to be, it nevertheless is, phenomenologically speaking, an *ontological reality, ensuing from and stimulating of an energy* dynamic for its affectively – or motivationally – propelled drive.

In the abstract paintings of John Day, Agnes Martin, and Geneviève Asse, to cite but three whose work overtly displays the motivational systems of PLAY and SEEKING, it is the synchrony of color, form, and texture that pleases the viewer as well as the creator, the viewer as co-creator, and without any hint of resemblance whatsoever to the recognizable. The same may be said of the most "modern" of choreographers, of composers and playwrights. Lacking recognizable shape, depth, and more, true abstraction is precisely that: what is removed from the known, from the identifiable. But there are those whose research in neuroaesthetics has led to the conclusion that such art, particularly abstract painting, is more anxiety-provoking than pleasure-inducing. There are those who claim such art to be less pleasing owing not only to a lack of the detectible, but the predictable. *Does Karl Friston's Free Energy Principle – his substantiation of the theory of predictive coding that shields us from surprise, from uncertainty, from chaos, and, indeed, from crisis – implicate a need for free energy minimization in the aesthetic experience?* Does "Friston's Law," as Solms calls it,[70] implicate aesthetic pleasure and displeasure in accordance with predictive coding? Does it implicate a potential for equilibration and its opposite owing to prediction accuracy and error in the domain of creativity? Is one to conceptualize some sort of dysregulation beyond the physiological in the context of the imaginative? It is to these and related questions that the following chapter is devoted.

Notes

1 Antonio Damasio, *The Strange Order of Things: Life, Feeling, and the Making of Cultures* (Vintage Books, 2018), 239.
2 Frank J. Sulloway, *Freud, Biologist of the Mind* (Basic Books, 1979).
3 François Ansermet and Pierre Magistretti, *Biology of Freedom: Neural Plasticity, Experience, and the Unconscious*, trans. Susan Fairfield (Other Press, 2007), 191.
4 Mark Solms, "Revision of Drive Theory," *JAPA* 69, no. 6 (2022): 1038.
5 Mark Solms, *The Only Cure: Freud and the Neuroscience of Mental Healing* (Weidenfeld & Nicholson, 2026).
6 H.W. Smith. *From Fish to Philosopher* (1953), cited in Jaak Pankesepp, *Affective Neuroscience* (Oxford University Press, 1998), 164.
7 Sigmund Freud, "Instincts and Their Vicissitudes," *Standard Edition*, vol. 14, 120.
8 Oliver Sacks, *A Leg to Stand On* (Simon & Schuster, 1984), 164. Cited by Solms, "Revision of Drive Theory," 1086–87.
9 Solms, "Revision of Drive Theory," 1086.
10 Sigmund Freud, "On Narcissism: An Introduction," *Standard Edition*, vol. 14, 78.
11 Mark Solms, "The Neurobiological Underpinnings of Psychoanalytic Theory and Therapy." In *Frontiers in Behavioral Neuroscience* 12, article 294 (2018): 8.
12 Mark Solms, "The Conscious Id," *Neuropsychoanalysis* 15, no. 1 (2013): 5–19. DOI: 10.1080/15294145.2013.10773711
13 Sigmund Freud, "Beyond the Pleasure Principle," *Standard Edition*, vol. 18, 17.
14 Mark Solms, "The Hard Problem of Consciousness and the Free Energy Principle," *Frontiers in Psychology* 9, article 2714 (2019): 7.
15 Gilbert Simondon, *L'Individuation psychique et collective* (Aubier, 1989), 223. In Taylor Adkins, "A Short List of Gilbert Simondon's Vocabulary," *Fractal Ontology*, 2007. https://fractalontology.wordpress.com/2007/11/28/a-short-list-of-gilbert-simondons-vocabulary/
16 Solms, "Revision of Drive Theory," 1033.
17 Solms, "Revision of Drive Theory," 1052.
18 Solms, "Revision of Drive Theory," 1086.
19 Solms, "The Neurobiological Underpinnings of Psychoanalytic Theory and Therapy," 5.
20 Karl Friston, "Is the Free-Energy Principle Neurocentric?," *Nature Reviews Neuroscience* 11 (2010): 605. doi:10.1038/nrn2787-c2
21 Karl Friston, "The Free-Energy Principle: A Unified Brain Theory?," *Nature Reviews Neuroscience* 11 (2010): 127–38. doi:10.1038/nrn2787
22 Solms, "Revision of Drive Theory," 1052.
23 See Solms, "Revision of Drive Theory," 1064.
24 Wikipedia: Theory of Constructed Emotion.
25 See Mark Solms, *The Hidden Spring: A Journey to the Source of Consciousness* (W.W. Norton, 2021), 236.
26 Tomohiro Ishizu and Semir Zeki, "Toward a Brain-Based Theory of Beauty," *PLOS ONE* 6, no. 7 (2011): e21852. doi:10.1371/journal.pone.0021852
27 Ishizu and Zeki, "Toward a Brain-Based Theory of Beauty," 9 (emphasis added).
28 Beatrice Sbriscia-Fioretti, Cristina Berchio, David Freedberg, Vittorio Gallese, and Maria Alessandra Umiltà, "ERP Modulation during Observation of Abstract Paintings by Franz Kline," *PLOS ONE* 8, no. 10 (2013): e75241. doi:10.1371/journal.pone.0075241
29 See Vittorio Gallese, "Visions of the Body: Embodied Simulation and Aesthetic Experience," *Aisthesis. Pratiche, linguaggi e saperi dell'estetico* 10, no. 1 (2017): 41–50. doi:10.13128/Aisthesis-20902

30 Mark Solms, "Empathy as Developmental Achievement: Beyond Embodied Simulation," in *Neuroscience and Critique*, ed. Jan De Vos and Ed Pluth (Routledge, 2016), 204–5.
31 Freud, "Beyond the Pleasure Principle," 17.
32 See Solms, "Revision of Drive Theory," 1053.
33 John Day, *John Day* (Tenth Avenue Editions, Inc., 1984), 27.
34 See Karl Lunde, Introduction to John Day, *John Day* (Tenth Avenue Editions, 1984), 21.
35 Day, cited in *John Day*, 21.
36 See Iian Michael Brunt, "One Day." https://issuu.com/artadvisorch/docs/one_day
37 Cited by Brunt, "One Day."
38 Cited by Brunt, "One Day."
39 See Brunt, "One Day."
40 See Brunt, "One Day."
41 See Jaak Panksepp. *Affective Neuroscience: The Foundations of Human and Animal Emotions* (Oxford University Press, 1998), 168.
42 Panksepp, *Affective Neuroscience: The Foundations of Human and Animal Emotions*, 281.
43 Solms, "The Hard Problem of Consciousness and the Free Energy Principle."
44 Sigmund Freud, "Psychopathic Characters on the Stage," *Standard Edition*, vol. 7, 305.
45 See Solms, *The Hidden Spring*, 236.
46 See Panksepp, *Affective Neuroscience: The Foundations of Human and Animal Emotions*, 168.
47 See, for example, Marc Malmdorf Andersen et al., "Play in Predictive Minds: A Cognitive Theory of Play," *Psychological Review*. June 16, 2022. doi:10.1037/rev0000369
48 Victoria Stevens, "To Think without Thinking: The Implications of Combinatory Play and the Creative Process for Neuroaesthetics," *American Journal of Play* 7, no. 1 (2014): 99, 100, 105, 107.
49 Angela Moorjani, "Genesis, Child's Play, and the Gaze of Silence: Samuel Beckett and Paul Klee," *Samuel Beckett Today/Aujourd'hui* 19 (2007): 187.
50 Oxford Languages (languages.oup.com).
51 Nancy Princenthal, *Agnes Martin: Her Life and Art* (Thames & Hudson, 2015), 90–91.
52 Princenthal, *Agnes Martin: Her Life and Art*, 243.
53 Britt-Marie Schiller, "Figurability in the Art of Louise Bourgeois," *American Imago* 81, no. 3 (2024): 306.
54 Panksepp, *Affective Neuroscience: The Foundations of Human and Animal Emotions*, 296.
55 Rosalind Krauss, "Grids," *October* 9 (Summer 1979): 54.
56 Krauss, "Grids," 58, 59.
57 Krauss, "Grids," 61.
58 Panksepp, *Affective Neuroscience: The Foundations of Human and Animal Emotions*, 164.
59 Panksepp, *Affective Neuroscience: The Foundations of Human and Animal Emotions*, 145.
60 Solms, "Revision of Drive Theory," 1086, 1067.
61 Maurice Merleau-Ponty, *Le Visible et l'Invisible* (Gallimard, 1964), 251.
62 Eric R. Kandel, *Reductionism in Art and Brain Science* (Columbia University Press, 2016), 5 (emphasis added).
63 Silvia Supervielle, "Le temps arrêté," in *Geneviève Asse* (Éditions Palantines, 2004), 16.

64 Supervielle, "Le temps arrêté," 16.
65 See Solms, *The Hidden Spring*, 35.
66 Solms, "Revision of Drive Theory," 1086.
67 Robin L. Carhart-Harris and Karl J. Friston, "The Default-Mode, Ego-Functions and Free-Energy: A Neurobiological account of Freudian Ideas," Brain (February 28, 2010): 1275. doi:10.1093/brain/awq010
68 See Panksepp, *Affective Neuroscience: The Foundations of Human and Animal Emotions*, 168.
69 Cited in Kandel, *Reductionism in Art and Brain Science*, 130.
70 Solms, *The Hidden Spring*, 177.

Chapter 3

Curiosity and the Crisis of Uncertainty

What do we do when we look at a work of art? We associate, we empathize, we relate... Or so one might be inclined to respond. But "Artworks are actually as dead as doornails," we recall once again Solms having said. Writing of the absence of subjectivity in an object of perception, such as the work of art, one cannot empathize, he reasoned. The possibility of empathic error is therefore non-existent in aesthetics: While it "is possible to misperceive the state of another mind," such misperception is not possible with the appreciation of, say, a still life or a landscape. Once again, "Who is to say whether or not a willow is weeping?"[1] Nevertheless, we look. But if we cannot truly empathize – not with a non-representational work and not with a figurative work, not even a portrait for there is no subjectivity there either – what is it we are doing when we look? Compassion is hardly possible when there is "no one" for whom to feel it. In the most abstract of paintings, there is nothing about which to feel compassionate, nothing (i.e., no one) within which to instill a feeling of understanding and sharing; not of sorrow, not of joy. And still, we look. And we take pleasure in such looking. Why?

"The Role of Surprisal in Aesthetic Experience"

As I previously aimed to show, the "pull forward," the "becoming" of mind, as attested to by Neubauer, Abrams, and Balzert and unwittingly confirmed by Solms with Panksepp and Friston by his side, is a developmental process that involves "discontinuities" as well as "continuities." This is less simple a notion than it might appear. Consider, once more, what the French philosopher Gilbert Simondon wrote: "In a theory of the phases of being, becoming is something other than an alteration or a succession of states comparable to a serial development. Becoming is in effect a perpetuated and renovated *resolution*, an incorporating resolution, *proceeding through crises*, such that *its sense is in its center, not at its origin or its end*."[2] In what do such "crises" consist and what have they to do with our experience of art?

From the perspective of predictive processing, as we saw in the preceding chapter, prediction serves homeostatic need. And the minimization of

DOI: 10.4324/9781003566755-4

uncertainty is the defense against prediction error, against the potential for homeostatic "crisis" resulting from the accumulation of such errors, the "crisis" of which computational neuroscientists exploring this existential terrain speak. Probability guides our behavior. And learning and memory help to ensure maximum certainty while correcting the inaccurate suppositions or conjectures, the wrongful "inferences" or errors of predictability. "Increasing uncertainty is bad; decreasing uncertainty is good," Solms often reminds us, reiterating the biological imperatives or governing factors of the MindBody's maintenance of wellbeing. It is this that leads him to claim that consciousness itself is definable as "*felt uncertainty*,"[3] for need implicates awareness of need, which is to say the feeling of need, and it is feeling which governs the reduction we seek. As he also says, however, "Given my definition of consciousness as felt uncertainty, it is [...] interesting to note the role of surprisal in aesthetic experience."[4]

"Interesting" indeed, for "surprisal" has everything to do with aesthetic experience insofar as learning and memory, the neurobiological supports of expectation, are continually disrupted by errors in expectation, whether in literature or visual art, music or other performance art, leading to the conclusion of some that "felt uncertainty" reigns. Accounting for a number of neurological and psychiatric disorders, with somatic and/or psychopathic symptoms, the Free Energy Principle points to uncertainty as the origin of stress and to the brain's use of various mechanisms to predict sensory input from the environment, to elude surprise (prediction error) and settle uncertainty. It points to the brain's production of what is in effect a system of coding, a system enciphering expectations (or "priors") that allow us to successfully predict. Minimizing error in prediction, as previously discussed, is thus a persistent primary goal in the everyday lives of all human beings, a goal attained through either of two means: a change in expectation or a change in action, in what is termed by theorists of predictive coding an alteration of "the predicted sensory inputs" or "active inference." Why, then, might artists yield to the dis-order of prediction error in their making of art? Why might artists, as the painter Robert Pepperell has asked, cultivate a resistance to prediction error minimization in themselves, in their art, in others?[5]

Writing of visual art within the cognitive neuroscientific frame, Sander Van de Cruys and Johan Wagemans argue against overly simplistic concepts "such as harmony, perceptual fluency, and the so-called good Gestalt" in favor of the prediction processing theory as derived from the Free Energy Principle.[6] They explore the "predictive coding approach of perception [which] holds that the brain actively anticipates upcoming sensory input rather than passively [registering] it." As they explain, "On the basis of prior experience, the brain actively makes predictions about what visual input to expect in the current context of stimulation." And prediction errors "are the mismatches between these predictions and the current input" or "incoming [...] evidence."[7] Linking prediction with emotion on the basis of the founding of predictive coding "on homeostasis and the vital maintenance functions of the body," they argue that "to understand aesthetic emotion (appreciation)," they must make this link explicit.[8] Focusing primarily on "perceptual features of art and only briefly [touching] upon content, which can, of course, induce a whole range of emotions, from very straightforward ones (as, for example, in paintings of nudes) to very complex ones (as in paintings portraying social settings)," the authors write of the "obstacles" that visual artists "repeatedly and deliberately create." Why? Their answer, simply put, is that the resulting prediction errors are not necessarily negatively experienced.[9] Their answer is that "negative affect, discrepancy, and disruption" are "important components in aesthetic appreciation" insofar as there is "progression from a state of more unpredictability to a state of less uncertainty" and therein the pleasure of the artwork is said to lie.[10]

Though their work and that of others working in this arena is rich and informative, it leads to two problematic conclusions. The first is that the paintings which most impress us are those "in which we can, with some labor, distinguish recognizable, predictable forms."[11] Is recognition, however, *really* a prerequisite for the maximum appreciation of art? What does this say of abstraction – the excising from the recognizable to exclude the representational – not only in painting, but in music, dance, theater, or literature?

Consider the work of composer John Cage, music in which what he called "intended sounds" are sometimes absent and silence is shown not to exist in as much as unintended sounds – some recognizable (a sneeze by a member of the audience, for example), but also many not – are, at times, part of the musical performance. Cage's provocative scores were certainly controversial, yet they were also among the most important, among the most highly valued, of twentieth-century American music. And, clearly, pleasure in Cage's work, as in a multitude of other of the more avant-garde composers, does not reside uniquely or even primarily in the return of a recognizable pattern following an unanticipated increase in unexpected "tones, beats or chords."[12]

Consider the choreography of Isadora Duncan or that of Mary Wigman. Their renunciation of classical ballet (from toe shoes and tutus to the arabesque and onward from there) left nothing to recognition or even expectation as all that existed prior was discarded. Consider the acceptance of men into the world of American dance. That and much more is owed Ted Shawn who, with Ruth St. Denis, led the way for many a renowned choreographer to follow: Martha Graham, José Limón, Merce Cunningham, Doris Humphrey, Charles Weidman, and Hanya Holm, to cite but a few. The human body was recognizable; its movements were decidedly not.

And what is to be said of the Impressionist, Post-Impressionist, Fauvist, Dadaist, Surrealist, Cubist, Abstract Expressionist, or other modernist movements in painting? What is to be said of what Mary Ann Caws, with reference to Dada, calls its "*energizing ambivalence*"? What Caws "claim[s] for the enduring quality of Dada" is precisely "the flexibility of ambiguity and ambivalence and unresolvedness."[13] This is not to say the recognizable is not a source of pleasure, but that the very purpose of Dada was, as Caws says, "to operate in just that field of things which we wouldn't notice were they not called to our attention by their irrational presence and then their convergence."[14] Does the absence of expectation reductive of ambiguous sensory input truly explain the reason for the negative response of early modern and avant-garde literary and visual art? Was there really so significant a negative response? Were any of these movements ever as underappreciated as these authors claim? There have been artists and, indeed, entire movements whose originality has been disdained if not worse. Fashions come and go as readily in the aesthetic arena as in any other. One has only to think of the Impressionists and the response they initially received as compared with where they later came to be. And then there is "demand for the new" that we associate with the young and the elders' "love of the old" as described by the Irish writer of fiction Joyce Cary in his consideration of social implications inherent in the "joy of discovery."[15] But the idea that "recognizable, predictable forms" are the *sine qua non* of a highly positive response to art, I would argue, is historically unjustifiable. "Another point about the present period," wrote the minimalist painter and creator of freestanding constructions Donald Judd in 1964, "is that it is not a decline from Abstract Expressionism; it is not an interregnum; it does not have inferior art. Although the present does not have any one of Pollock's profundity – too many of the artists are too young – there are more good artists. The amount of good work is amazing. There is plenty of mediocre art, but there always is."[16] Similarly, the preeminent critic Hilton Kramer defended the "special strength" of non-figurative painting, its "audacity," its "brute visual power" which, he claimed, "other styles are powerless to match."[17] Some, like Rothko, bemoaned the early reception of his work. But great celebration of the painter's color field paintings, his association with Abstract Expressionism, was not long in coming.

Ladislav Kesner is another who has elegantly incorporated into the neurocognitive frame of prediction the psychological and subjective dimensions associated with it and accounted for cultural implications relative to aesthetic experience.[18] He, too, defines the appeal of the prediction coding account, incontestable in the behavioral context, but which he situates in that of the furthering of empirical studies of images and perceptions and the psychological understanding of art and its history. It is important to note that Kesner acknowledges the dynamic nature of the encounter of the beholder with the artwork. It is important to note that he recognizes how the prediction coding account serves as a scientific support of certain philosophical elucidations of aesthetic experience, such as the hermeneutic studies of philosophers like Hans-Georg Gadamer, which is to say that he stresses the potential for greater interdisciplinary dialogue with, if not the reliance of the predictive coding perspective upon, other explanatory frameworks. It is significant that he stops short of situating the minimization of uncertainty, of unpredictability, at the antipodes of the ontology of art.

Yet Kesner, as well, writes of the "resistance and aversion to contemporaneous art [that] have been constant features of the development of modern art since its inception."[19] He, too, pursues cognitive components inherent within a supposed repugnance, an antipathy he relates to cultural determinants and an inability to identify objects in visual images. And this, once again, is where, to my way of thinking, things go terribly wrong. While the claim of "aversion" is historically accurate to a degree (though I would venture that it was not as widespread and historically longstanding as Kesner claims), identification, "knowing" in this way what one is viewing, is by no means prerequisite to aesthetic pleasure. Rather, it is *in the very drive to know* (sensorially or cerebrally), which is to say *in curiosity itself*, in *engaging proactively with uncertainty*, in SEEKING – *and the creativity it impels* – that pleasure is to be found. While "being curious is not a sufficient condition for creativity," as the astrophysicist Mario Livio has remarked, "Curiosity does appear [...] to be a *necessary* condition for creativity."[20] And whether viewed as the "diversion of sexual instinctual forces from sexual aims," as Freud defined sublimation,[21] or as epistemically pleasurable unto itself, it is in the role played by curiosity, by SEEKING, in the epistemophilic dimension of this emotional drive, that pleasure resides. It is the quest itself as opposed to the verification of expected results that looms large in modern art, particularly in the paintings of Abstract Expressionism, I would argue. This is not to say that pleasure associated with the reduction of prediction error is insignificant. Indeed, SEEKING, as the so-called "default" drive, the only emotional drive preemptively engaged with uncertainty, secures prediction where "crisis" is the risk of surprise. Yet the disregard for the pleasure residing within the very state of being curious is challenging.

The second conclusion similarly arises from the predictive processing theory, a theory whose application to aesthetic experience appears valid though conclusions too readily drawn from it may in themselves be highly questionable: From the learning-based perspective of predictive coding, Van de Cruys, along with Jo Bervoets and Agnes Moors, deduces that "frequent engagement with a piece of art or music detract[s] from its emotionality [...], suggesting that we are often chasing an experience we cannot fully relive when revisiting the same artwork."[22] This is a stunning supposition, especially for the ease with which it may be experientially refuted.

If homeostasis is to be seen as the fundamental objective in accordance with which drives operate, it is also to be said that the body as such is not necessarily the source of all identifiable drives, as Panksepp showed. There is a distinction to be made between bodily drives, such as the need for nourishment, and emotional drives, like that experienced by the giver of care. Yet, as we saw in Chapter Two, for Solms as for Panksepp, both kinds of drive are allied with affect. And the searching, the foraging behavior of SEEKING, not pleasurable in aesthetic experience simply as a function of curiosity understood as the means to a reprieve from the unexpected but, as Solms suggests, "an 'appetitive' affect," is an affect *pleasurable in and of itself*.[23] In an 1882 letter to his brother, Van Gogh reiterated a statement he had previously made elsewhere: "'I am an artist'" and "these words connote, 'Always seeking without absolutely, finding.'"[24] His terms could not have been more apt, for SEEKING is what the artist does. It is also what the reader, listener, or spectator does as well. As Samuel Beckett wrote, "Art has always been this – pure interrogation, rhetorical question less the rhetoric."[25]

Curiosity, then, in the context of aesthetic experience arises from surprisal. It is what emanates from the unexpected and leads to the imaginative – which is to say creative – updating of erroneous expectation or prediction error. And it adds to the pleasure of looking, listening, and reading involving some notion of "beauty." But the maximum of aesthetic appreciation, I would argue, is *neither to be reductively defined as the pleasure emanating from the negative response to uncertainty nor limited to the initial encounter with the work of art*.

To speak of the crisis of uncertainty is to speak of the crisis of creativity that flows from within it, a crisis not to be confused either with a lack of inspiration or with the lack of imagination said by some to stem from creativity as a skill, learnable and performable as "procedural knowledge," as Lisa Barrett Feldman refers to it, and originating in conceptualization.[26] "'Conception' cannot precede 'execution,'" as Maurice Merleau-Ponty so rightly said of artistic imagination.[27] Neurobiologically speaking, the crisis of creativity stems from that of equilibration and survival, from the crisis of uncertainty. And when considered in the context of aesthetics, it resides in the emotional capacity to withstand the instability, the insecurity, that creativity demands of the creator, the "deformation" unleashed by the creative energy, the force of the creative process. What is the securing of information in the aesthetic realm, the quest that is curiosity, if not the state of being in-formation, itself a perilous venture? As Evelyne Grossman writes, "A risk [...] is involved in the very movement of every creation, that of the calcification, the progressive petrification of the processes at play. It is probably necessary to be gifted with an extraordinarily plastic and malleable drive energy to resist the solidifications in which the creative processes always threaten to set themselves."[28]

Like SEEKING, the neural source of curiosity and creativity, CARE is another emotional system identified by Panksepp as associated with curiosity and pleasurable in and of itself. By way of this foundational system of the brain, we also arrive at some understanding of the appeal of certain works of art over others. CARE pertains, of course and above all, to nurturance (to parental behavior and that of mothers, in particular, due to the brain circuits and chemistry involved). But nurturance is not the only manifestation of this basic operating system. In an interview for *The New York Times*, cellist Yo Yo Ma spoke of his job as a musician, his responsibility of ensuring that no one is more important in the room than the listener. What matters, he explained, is "caring" about where one is and why and, expounding upon CARE in music, he described it as an energy that bonds human beings. In uniting people, that energy, that sound moving air molecules, is an acknowledgment of another's being, their presence, and it is this that brings happiness to Ma and to others, as he put it.[29]

With regard to the pleasure of music – how it connects with us emotionally, makes meaning in the absence of words, and stimulates us to move – Panksepp and Colwyn Trevarthen have shown that our appreciation of rhythm and our engagement with it derive from subcortical emotional systems activating the cerebral hemispheres.[30] Challenging the hierarchy of cognitive versus affective – and, even more fundamentally, epistemic versus ontological – explanations in favor of their interrelation, they have explored the psychobiology of music to elucidate the very meaning of meaning itself. The significance of the release of dopamine, the neurotransmitter known to be activated by the hearing of pleasurable music – as by maternal attachment, by CARE – is certainly relevant to this interrelation, to the interconnection between the epistemic and ontological, between knowing and being. This consideration of affect as implicated in the pleasures of curiosity, creativity, and care is in no way meant to diminish the significant contribution of prediction and the associated reduction of uncertainty as regards aesthetics. To be sure, much is to be said of the neural circuitry and its role in guiding our affective response to music. Citing the cortical circuits that foster our making of predictions, Robert J. Zatorre and Valorie N. Salimpoor have described the accumulation of information over time, the creation of models deriving from one's cultural milieu and their facilitating of the listener's comprehension of music subsequently heard.[31] At the same time, however, it bears repeating that the conclusions referred to above – namely, that recognition is requisite to maximum aesthetic pleasure and that the degree of emotional pleasure is necessarily limited in the re-viewing of a visual artwork – fall demonstrably short.

Among others who have contributed significantly to neuroaesthetics, to our understanding of the neural correlates of the appreciation of art, is Edward Vessel. Proposing that certain artworks have greater appeal owing to the relevance of the work to the viewer's, reader's, or listener's sense of self, Vessel, with G. Gabrielle Starr and Nava Rubin, regards as integral to aesthetic experience the Default Mode Network (DMN), that region of the brain activated introspectively when at rest:

> We propose that certain artworks can "resonate" with an individual's sense of self in a manner that has well-defined physiological correlates and consequences: the neural representations of those external stimuli obtain access to the neural substrates and processes concerned with the self – namely, to regions of the DMN. This access, which other external stimuli normally do not obtain, allows the representation of the artwork to interact with the neural processes related to the self, affect them, and possibly even be incorporated into them (i.e., into the future, evolving representation of self).[32]

Insofar as the "resonance" in question is said to be not only self-referential but even, at times, "bidirectional" – with "externally-directed ('task-positive') brain networks" detecting "a certain 'harmony' between the external world and our internal representation of the self – allowing the two systems to co-activate, interact, influence and reshape each other,"[33] their understanding of aesthetic *pleasure* becomes clearer: It resides in harmony not only as the *absence* of dissonance, of incompatibility, of disorder, and the unexpectable, but as the *presence* of the self as known, a dimension the authors deem, when particularly intense, "thrillingly bidirectional":

> [N]ot only does the perceiver feel as if they understand the artwork, but there is a sense that the artwork "understands" the perceiver, expressing one's own innermost thoughts, feelings, or values. The latter sense points to the possibility that it is the artist, not the artwork, who has understood something deep about the perceiver's experience; hence the intensely personal connection felt by many people toward favorite artists who are, after all, strangers to them.[34]

This emphasis on the subjective is very much in keeping with the variability of one's response to art as dependent upon one's emotional state at the time of viewing. Like the conclusions noted above, however, the idea that the most appreciated of artworks are those in which there resides a resonance with the sense of self is also problematic given the fundamental question that subtends it – the meaning of "bidirectional," the meaning of intersubjective, in the absence of a subject – to which I will return shortly.

If Solms, like Freud, situates development on the trajectory of maturation of the ego, the trajectory that emanates from the connection between psyche and soma and follows from learning by experience, he also distinguishes himself from Freud, as we have seen, by revising the classical notion of drive in accordance with what he considers its essence: the subjectivity of feeling.[35] Like Neubauer, Abrams, and Balzert, he defines the learning through experience that constitutes the "inherent impetus," the "pull forward" (Abrams' terms), though with a different emphasis and vocabulary. Writing of affect as "a category which contains emotional tone, mood, and emotions" (one of twelve categories comprising their organization of data), the authors of the manuscript discussed in Chapter One stress *the dispositional component of affect*, the dominant biological element influential (even seminal) in affect development. And, in considering the genetic and other biological factors, they offer a view of affect that, in its striking concordance with Solms' revision of drive theory, obliges us to consider just how extensive is the association between the awareness of one's own subjective feelings and the learning stimulated by the unexpected. In the context of art, it is this that defines "the role of surprisal in aesthetic experience."

This is hardly to say that imagining, creating, is solely constituted by the avoidance of crisis (understood not in the sense of catastrophe, in the sense of calamity as used colloquially, or even in the physiological sense, but in the sense of the turmoil, the confusion, the instability, turbulence, and consequent stress of uncertainty) or that the biological imperative is entirely determinative. It *is* to say that the generation of curiosity from which creativity ensues, that the generation of curiosity by the energic emotional drive system of SEEKING, like those of PLAY and CARE, is *conjoined with conscious awareness of feeling*. How significant it is to recognize this in the context of the appreciation of art. And how significant it is to recognize the value of memory and learning as well, *the value of predictive processing in the appreciation of art*. An additional problem arises, however, when the interrelation between the epistemology and ontology of art are substantially diminished if not entirely ignored. A problem arises, in other words, when subjective experience is discounted. To cite Mark Rothko once again, "A painting is not a picture of an experience. It is an experience."[36] Just as a theatrical performance is not a re-presentation, but an actuality, a painting, like the poem or novel, "is not *about* something; *it is that something itself*," as Samuel Beckett similarly claimed when writing of James Joyce.[37] And to the extent that art is deemed embedded in the conceptual accounts offered by cognitive neuroscience, it loses existential and thereby ontological ground. I will return to this in the following chapter, but the fundamental question referred to but a moment ago requires consideration first.

Intersubjectivity in the Absence of a Subject

What is the meaning of intersubjectivity if there is no subject in the work of art? Questioning the meaning of intersubjectivity in the absence of a subject, in art said to be "a little bit of nothing" as the Abstract Expressionist Larry Rivers put it, "not real" as Solms has said, is to pose a question seemingly so concrete as to be worthy only of being dismissed. But a problem does arise when the interrelation between the curiosity involved in the making and viewing of art – the interrelation between the epistemophilic drive stimulating the creativity of any artist or engaged viewer – and the ontology of art is disregarded. A problem does arise when subjectivity in aesthetic experience is ignored. Is this subjectivity, however, reducible to an "intercorporeal" view of such experience, to a view of the aesthetic as a "mediated form of intersubjectivity" as Vittorio Gallese, David Freedberg, and others would have it?[38]

As previously noted, and is well-known, Gallese has offered much in the way of defining aesthetic experience. Basing his assessment on the theoretical account of embodied simulation, on the role of empathy as supported by research on mirror neurons, he has made an invaluable contribution to the appreciation of art, whether visual, literary, or performative. While accounts of simulation theory – some focusing on what is known as low-level simulation (the attribution of mental states to others) and some on its counterpart, high-level simulation (the generation of imaginative states) – are numerous, there are those, however, who dispute the simulation theory of empathy whatever the approach. Philosopher Shaun Gallagher has impressively defined several problems associated with neural simulation accounts and substituted an explanation of empathy having everything to do with a

Figure 3.1 Mark Rothko (American, born Daugavpils, Russia (now Latvia), 1903–1970), *Orange and Yellow*, 1956. Oil on canvas. 91 x 71 inches (231.14 x 180.34 cm). Collection Buffalo AKG Art Museum. Gift of Seymour H. Knox, Jr., 1956 (K1956:8). © Kate Rothko Prizel & Christopher Rothko / Artists Rights Society (ARS), New York. Photo: Brenda Bieger, Buffalo AKG Art Museum.

contextualization of the motivation and plight of the other as a way around those problems. If Solms signals the absence of a subject in the artwork with whom to empathize and deems embodied simulation more a matter of reflection, a reflexive instrument not necessarily unrelated to but not the instrument of empathy, Gallagher questions simulation as an explanation of empathy to the extent that narrative contextualization and interaction are lacking. Communication, understanding, evaluation and more are required, as he sees it, for the "narrative practice" irreducible to processes of cognition and requisite to empathy. Rejecting the notion that "understanding another person's action relies on a neural mechanism that matches the observed behavior with a behavior that the observer could execute," Gallagher comes no closer than Solms to accepting the idea that simulation explains empathy.[39]

While it is not my intention to explore simulation theory here, I will simply make mention of Gallese's exploration of the corporeal engagement with art, the bodily responses felt by the viewer said to underlie empathic response, as discussed by him and art historian David Freedberg in "Motion, Emotion and Empathy in Esthetic Experience." For, unlike others who have sought to describe the pleasurable response to art based on what they refer to as the "psychophysical and neurocognitive" workings of the visual components of the brain, the authors of this paper, in specifying those mechanisms said to give rise to the empathic intensity of images, raise questions particularly relevant to what I will argue here. They cite sculptures and paintings (such as one by Michelangelo exhibiting the sense of exertion and another by Goya showing physical injury) which figure what is said to incite empathic response. At the same time, they stress that such response, the result of bodily engagement with the work, is not limited to any sort of figuration, but similarly stimulated by the gestural movement of the artist's hand ("brushmarks or paint drippings") and the intentionality of the artist in non-figurative art as well. Claiming that mirroring mechanisms – which may be precognitive (or not necessarily contingent upon cognitively informed perception) – are requisite to aesthetic appreciation, they go so far as to suggest that simulated embodiment informs artistic skill. This is to say that, insofar as artists "more or less successfully make conscious and unconscious use of body knowledge" to stimulate certain kinds of emotional and bodily responses, a distinct role for simulated embodiment is said to be part of the creation as well as the reception of the artwork. Cited in this regard are the cut canvases of Lucio Fontana "where sight of the slashed painting invites a sense of empathetic movement that seems to coincide with the gesture felt to have produced the tear."[40]

Gallese has elsewhere spoken of the brain's sensory-motor system's embodiment of abstract concepts – of linguistic constructions in the literary text, for example – and other not manifestly visual forms of expression.[41] But it is in this essay that he and Freedberg name Merleau-Ponty as another in whose work one finds significant recognition of the association of painting and sculpture with motoric arousal. And it is with the empathic dimension of that association that I would both disagree and base what follows on the reasons for my disagreement. Indeed, Merleau-Ponty, a phenomenologist who has had great influence on the thinking of philosophers and aestheticians alike, is clearly not one whose work I find consonant with the "felt bodily imitation of the implied actions of the artist" and other such notions as put forth by Freedberg and Gallese.[42] When his essay "Cézanne's Doubt" appeared in 1945, this mastermind of phenomenology was already dedicated to what he called "the indivisible whole": "[T]he world is a mass without gaps, a system of colors across which the receding perspective, the outlines, angles, and curves are inscribed like lines of force; the spatial structure vibrates as it is formed."[43] Such "lines of force," I would add if somewhat parenthetically, are the very lines to which PLAY – as well as SEEKING, with its correlation to curiosity and the need to know – give form. Galen Johnson has put it thus: "Being itself, for Merleau-Ponty [...], is imbued with a kind of energy, longing, desire or *conatus*."[44]

But the point is this: For Merleau-Ponty, expressing the world, as is the painter's wont, is not about dichotomizing or distinguishing subject from object, a dichotomy implicit in embodied simulation. Subject and object for Merleau-Ponty are, in fact, the very antithesis of such dichotomizing: "[T]he seer," as Johnson would explain of the philosopher's writing on painting, "is caught up in the midst of the visible, [...] in order to see, the seer must in turn be capable of being seen."[45] Merleau-Ponty could not have stated it more clearly: "The lived object is not rediscovered or constructed on the basis of the contributions of the senses; rather, it presents itself to us from the start as the center from which these contributions radiate. We *see* the depth, the smoothness, the softness, the hardness of objects; Cézanne even claimed that we see their odor."[46] Cézanne exemplifies, as it is the philosopher's purpose to show, the challenge posed to subject-object division by the depiction of matter *as it takes form through vision*, through the very practice of seeing by artist and viewer alike. For painting "evokes nothing," Merleau-Ponty wrote in his celebrated essay "Eye and Mind"; rather, it "gives visible existence to what profane vision believes to be invisible; thanks to it we do not need a 'muscular sense' in order to possess the voluminosity of the world."[47]

Interestingly, this unity to which the philosopher subscribes does not deny the notion of embodiment; in fact, it subscribes to it: "[T]he interrogation of painting [...] looks toward this secret and feverish genesis of things in our body."[48] Yet it is relegated to the status of an appendage of the ontological as captured by art maker and viewer: "This voracious vision, reaching beyond the 'visual givens,' opens upon a texture of Being of which *the discrete sensorial messages are only the punctuations or the caesurae*."[49] Like the "reversibility of subject and object" felt by all – *one hand touching the other is felt by the first hand as well as the second*, Johnson reminds us – such is vision. To see, seers must themselves be seeable, a reality not empathic, but ontological; a reality "exemplified in our own bodies," as Johnson writes, "as a fundamental manifestation of Being."[50] Less a feeling (empathy) emanating from brain physiology than a melding of self with the visible world – a "lending" of the body to the world, as Merleau-Ponty famously described the act of making art[51] – painting reveals an exchange that may be reversed but a moment later, a reversibility more chiasmic, more intertwining, than divisive and thereby potentially empathic. And it is this attribute of the ontological, this chiasmatic relation of seer with seen (justifying the dual-aspect monism referred to regarding consciousness in Chapter One and about which more later), that brings us yet closer to the interplay of curiosity and the crisis of uncertainty.

In "Cézanne's Doubt," Merleau-Ponty, writing of the painter's rapidly transitioning post-Impressionist art, deemed it "paradoxical," for Cézanne was said to be "pursuing reality without giving up the sensuous surface, with no other guide than the immediate impression of nature, without following the contours, with no outline to enclose the color, with no perspectival or pictorial arrangement." Cézanne's pursuit of reality, "while denying himself the means to attain it," was said to be responsible for the distortions prevailing in his art between 1870 and 1890. "Cups and saucers on a table seen from the side should be elliptical, but Cézanne paints the two ends of the ellipse swollen and expanded," Merleau-Ponty wrote. Cézanne, in a word, was said to be "abandoning himself to *the chaos of sensation*."[52]

This upsetting of objects and suggesting of illusions, lack of frame for color, and absence of graphic arrangement is what caused another Post-Impressionist painter, Emile Bernard, to claim Cézanne "'submerged his paintings in ignorance and his mind in shadows.'" "But one cannot really judge his painting this way," counters Merleau-Ponty, "except by closing [...] one's eyes to what he painted."[53] Challenging dichotomies, moreover, those of sensation and judgment, seeing and thinking, nature and composition, primitive and traditional, was the painter's intent, and what Merleau-Ponty suggested was that viewers sensitize themselves to the meaning of the painting alone, a meaning which escaped these oppositions and that between feeling and thinking as well. Cézanne, Merleau-Ponty determined, "did not think he had to choose between feeling and thought, as if he were deciding between *chaos and order*."[54]

What he describes as "Cézanne's uncertainty,"[55] moreover, is explained by Merleau-Ponty not in terms of the painter's psyche (though he does not discard its contribution), but by his desire to create in such a way that *expression* in and of itself, the "lived perspective,"[56] is experienced by the viewer as constituting the art. Cézanne "did not want to separate the stable things which we see and the shifting way in which they appear; he wanted to depict matter *as it takes on form*, the birth of order through spontaneous organization."[57]

This capturing of vision, this securing of the experiential, of the actuality of perception, is, of course, what inspired the mid-to-late 19th-century Impressionists to make art at different moments in the daily cycle of time as the impact of light on the exterior evolved. It was the way they, and all Modernist painters, in a sense, demonstrated variations in perception, disparities in observation and awareness stemming from the personal. "The painter lives in fascination," Merleau-Ponty would write, and it was this fascination, this curiosity, that impelled the painter to make art revealing as much of the seer as the seen, art exposing the feeling, the

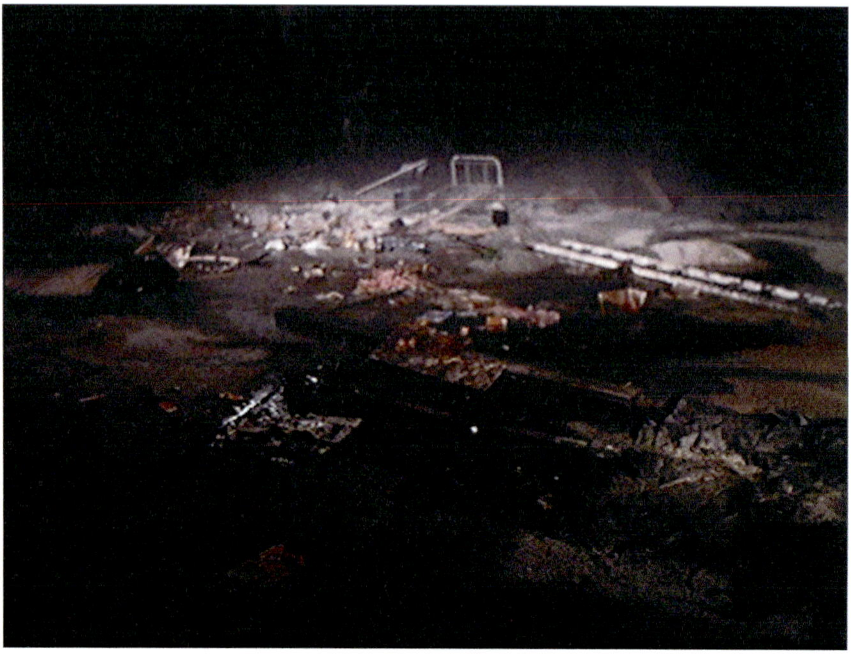

Figure 3.2 Samuel Beckett, *Breath* (1969). Curran-Moseid 1988

sensitivity, of each hand at it touches the other.[58] It was not the exterior, but the interrelation of the external with the internal that was painted. "'The landscape thinks itself in me […] and I am its consciousness,'" Merleau-Ponty quoted Cézanne as saying.[59] This abstraction of meaning from the exterior with a concomitant constitution of interior meaning would find its way into the modernist aesthetic more generally in the years to come, not only in painting but in other forms of art as well.

In Samuel Beckett's *Breath* (first performed in 1969), for example, as in other of his writings for the theater, the playwright/novelist/poet aimed to reveal consciousness beyond its capacity for conceptualization. Long concerned with the limits of language as a modality of expression and with those of action as a means of achievement, Beckett created this play – a theater piece lasting but approximately 35 seconds, having no dialogue revealing emotions with which to empathize and no personalities with which to identify; in fact, a play with no characters at all – to afford visualization of life not conceptually or even emotionally comprehensible, yet lived. Like the final words of his 1953 novel *The Unnamable* – "I can't go on, I'll go on" – which puts existence itself in high relief, *Breath* captures in two identical cries of a newborn, cries fused with a "slow increase" and "decrease of light," the experience of being conscious, aware, alive. What the play offers is purity of mind and thereby of feeling (no matter how ambiguous or abstract) and it does so by virtue of the lack of figuration of any living being. What the play offers is the lack of certainty of any kind: which is to say crisis. Yet there is this: a "stage littered with miscellaneous rubbish."[60] Just what is the relation of that setting to the disembodied cries? Just what kind of visual impression is made upon the viewer who hears the source of existential pain but does not bear visual witness to anything but scattered waste? Absent the human figure, however audible, subjectivity in this play is denied, but the expression of deep emotion in the two cries of the infant renders subjectivity at the same time exceedingly present. The result is not a dichotomous presence and absence, but a congruence, the *Dasein* (or "being there") of which Martin Heidegger wrote. This yielding of the self to the non-self, this capitulation to disembodiment, is achieved, if paradoxically, by emptiness as a presence in itself. Presence in this play, in other words, *is* by virtue of its material absence,[61] and presence and absence play ("PLAY") with one another here as in so many other of Beckett's writings as well.

The act of writing, in fact, serves as an example of a similar irony in as much as it was a means for Beckett of disarticulating as much as articulating. Considering Beckett's final work, the poem entitled "What Is the Word" written when he was recovering from aphasia (the result of an ill-defined neurological disorder), Laura Salisbury has said the following: "If to be is to be perceived, or perhaps if to be is also to be a perceiving subject that can order perceptions into a sense of 'mine', then 'What Is the Word' disarticulates the coherence of such speaking/perceiving beings. Nevertheless, some kind of reconfigured and dislocated subject does persist in the poem." Writing of a "subjectless poem" and of "subjectless seeing," she questions "what is left of a perceiving being [...] thrown amidst a thickened and resistant material world that will not yield to either naming or comprehension, as language becomes a crust of material signifiers that occludes representation." Noting that "Words are no longer perceptible and perfected figures or Gestalts, standing out in proud relief against a ground of meaningless noise," she describes Beckett's use of language as "a material, opaque surface upon which figure and ground relentlessly convert into one another. In 'What Is the Word', writing has indeed become all surface, an unfolding of linguistic permutation that explicitly occludes the hallucination of an essential or self-present meaning humming behind the material marks on the surface of the page."[62]

Absence versus awareness of the void, of the vacuum or the emptiness of the human condition as depicted by the playwrights of the Theater of the Absurd, are not, however, conflated by Beckett.[63] It is precisely recognition of their distinction and the interplay between them that his 1972 play *Not I* puts fully center stage by having the only character, no more than a mouth (aptly named, as mentioned previously, Mouth), verbalize much with which to empathize but, at the same time, be no one with whom to do so.

In this work, unlike in *Breath*, presence is figured, if only as an empty signifier, a facial feature no more than a vacuum. And yet, despite its visually conveying nothing but emptiness, *it is there*, so much so in fact that the entire focus of this monologue is Mouth's refutation of her very self, a refutation that takes the form

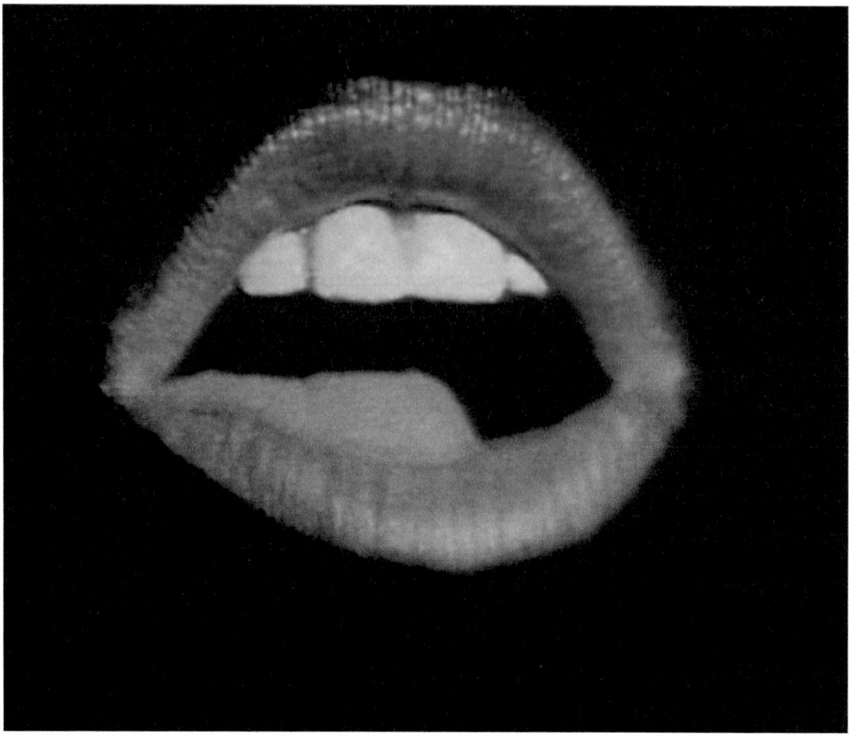

Figure 3.3 Samuel Beckett, *Not I*, 1972 (1977) Single-channel video, b/w, sound, 11 min 52 s MACBA Collection. MACBA Consortium

of a "vehement refusal to relinquish [the] third person" (as indicated by Beckett's preliminary note to the play[64]). By remaining steadfastly connected to "she," Mouth defines what remains when the first person rejects her own identity: nothing. Here again, it is within the play of presence and absence – framed in this work by the complexity, the incomprehensibility even, of what is recounted by the voice – that the spectator seeks to understand, to conceptualize, what cannot be conceptualized: existence itself. It is not for nothing that Beckett's late play *What Where* (which premiered in 1983) nears its end as follows:

> Time passes.
> That is all.
> Make sense who may.[65]

The point is that *dis*embodiment, literally and metaphorically, is where this writer's attention most often lies, in his novels as in the plays, much as it does in the art of the most highly abstract painters, which throws into question the notion of empathy as embodied simulation and even prediction error minimization as the primary source of pleasure in aesthetic experience. Why might artists, as I previously asked, yield to the disorder of prediction error? Why might they cultivate a resistance to prediction error minimization in themselves, in their art, in others? It is for what the British critic Martin Esslin described in 1961 as "the starting point of a new kind of consciousness," one that "faces the mystery and terror of the human condition in the exhilaration of a new-found freedom." As Esslin explains with regard to Beckett's work in its entirety, it "can be seen as a search for the reality that lies beyond mere reasoning in conceptual terms." And with regard to Beckett's theater, "it is possible to bypass the stage of conceptual thinking altogether, as an abstract painting bypasses the stage of the recognition of natural objects."[66]

Devoid of character, plot, and meaningful (in the sense of narratively consequential) dialogue, Beckett's plays, like his novels and the work of many a modernist writer, were and remain highly appreciated *precisely for their ambiguity*, though some in cognitive neuroscience would dispute such a claim. What Pepperell calls "visual indeterminacy," and to which I would add semantic indeterminacy, need not be reduced for uncertainty, or the anticipation of its reduction, to produce pleasure insofar as curiosity, fascination, as I have already stressed, is in itself pleasurable and, I would add, not merely pleasurable but often exhilarating. Many are those who prefer the indeterminate for reasons that go beyond both anticipation of uncertainty minimization and the arousal intrinsic to seeking, inherent within the quest. As Pepperell suggests of prediction errors, "maximizing these errors, within certain bounds, can effectively heighten one's sense of existence." In agreement with a statement made by the British painter Bridget Riley – namely, that "[p]erception constitutes our awareness of what it is to be human, indeed what it is to be alive" – he reasons that if "being aware is what it is to feel alive, and if highly salient prediction errors are marked by heightened state of awareness, then maximizing these errors, within certain bounds, can effectively heighten one sense of existence. In other words, the multifarious, contradictory, paradoxical, and ideological states of mind produced in a person when they look intensely at the world, or at a powerful work of art, make us alive to the world." The resolution of ambiguity, on the one hand, and the pursuit of information in and of itself, on the other, are undeniably inducive of pleasure. But the interaction of our comprehending minds with both our perceiving bodies and the world may be constitutive of pleasure such that the desire for the indeterminate, the ambiguous, rules.[67]

In a 1964 essay entitled "The 'Crisis' of Abstract Art," the renowned art critic Clement Greenberg cited a number of French writers who, in a mimeographed list of statements in French and English prepared by the now defunct monthly magazine *Preuves*, addressed what they saw as the "crisis" of painting, of the painting known as the "informel" – literally, without form – or Abstract Expressionism. Greenberg found nothing new in this so-called "crisis," locating the catastrophe in the domain of art criticism rather than in the art itself. For, interestingly, he finds no such thing as formlessness in the painting of this era and he considers the so-called "crisis" of abstraction to concern not an absence of form, a notion he rightly claims to be meaningless (and about which more in Chapter Four), but the exhaustion of the kind of art he refers to as "Painterly Abstraction." More specifically, the second generation of this art making, Greenberg determined, produced art not formless but formulaic; art not authentic but false and uninspired.

In "The Crisis of the Easel Picture" from 1948, Greenberg had already described a critical state of painting, one in which uniformity was the operative motif. "The very notion of uniformity is antiaesthetic," he disparagingly proclaimed. "Yet many 'all-over' pictures seem to succeed precisely by virtue of their uniformity, their sheer monotony. The dissolution of the pictorial into sheer texture, into apparently sheer sensation, into an accumulation of repetitions, seems to speak for and answer something profound in contemporary sensibility."[68] What was that sensibility and why did these "all-over pictures" succeed? On the one hand, what Greenberg was reproaching was the commercialism, the financial interest to which art was falling prey. On the other, he was anticipating what was to follow: the perceptual ambiguity and semantic indeterminacy of the Expressionism to come. I bring Greenberg into this consideration of the crisis of uncertainty because his view of the New York School (those artists painting in New York City in the mid-twentieth century) exemplifies the idea that it is that very ambiguity itself that affords pleasure in abstract art.

To return, however, to the neuroscience that is increasingly informing explorations of aesthetic experience, sometimes with validity and sometimes without, or so I would argue, Anil Seth is one who has succeeded in describing the relation between interoceptive and exteroceptive inference, the perception of the internal world by autonomic or visceral reflexes and that of the external world by sensory input. Seth has concluded not only as to the inevitable shaping of emotional response by exteroceptive contextualization, but "that perceptual scenes that evoke interoceptive predictions will always be affectively coloured."[69] Together with Karl Friston he has offered a review of the recent "re-conceptualization" of interoception and its implications for the experiencing of emotion as well as of selfhood to arrive, perhaps most significantly for my objective here, at the reversal of the cartesian cogito.[70] "I am therefore I think": What is the relation of that dictum to the "I feel therefore I am" with which the first chapter of this book began?

Claudia Muth, along with Marius Hans Raab and Claus-Christian Carbon, has offered a way into an answer in describing how perception as impacted by the environmental context of viewing is comparable to how "person-related factors like personality, experience, expertise and mood" bear upon the viewing experience. The intricacy of the work itself is an additional perspective from which to consider the encounter contributing to the "realm of psycho-aesthetics" with which they are concerned. Each of these perceptual processes "is an attempt to construct semantic stability involving person- as well as context-related factors rather than a passive registration of determinate meanings." Artists may play, they note, with violating "perceptual habits as well as the context of art perception itself." But here is the point: "Such 'prediction errors' should lead to negative affect because 'they signal that there is something wrong with the mental model we use to generate the predictions,'" as Van de Cruys and Wagemans have claimed. Yet various theoretical accounts explain "how the encounter with such displeasing, highly arousing deviations of stimulations from predictions is still able to ultimately evoke pleasure in the perceiver." Enjoyment may emanate not only from the diminution of uncertainty, from the easy processing of objects, from humor "induced by a *resolution* of incongruity," and the like. "Furthermore," as Muth et al. convincingly proclaim, "not every person might react to the mechanisms of increased predictability of Aesthetic Aha in the same way: for instance, people differ in their (in)tolerance of ambiguity [...] and this seems to influence the appreciation of ambiguity in art." Depending upon mood, moreover, the same work of art may affect the same person in different ways at different times.[71]

While the degree of pleasure depends upon the viewer or reader – their tolerance of ambiguity, their mood at the time of the encounter with the work in question, to say nothing of their psychology in a more general sense – it is important to remember that it is the *defiance* of abstract expression that evokes the response. It is the *challenge* posed by the surprisal that is of significance when one considers the phenomenology of the aesthetic encounter. Without a subject posing that challenge, however, one must ask just *how the sensory system*, whatever the mode of perception, *is responsible for stimulating the drives* considered in the previous chapter: PLAY and SEEKING, primarily. For this is precisely where the paths of those exploring this terrain diverge.

With some continuing to focus primarily or entirely on the centrality of the ocular, others on the dialectic of the Merleau-Pontyian chiasmus, and still others on the neural activation of embodied simulation à la Gallese, it is the intersection of the neurobiological with the psychoanalytic – which is to say, the neuropsychoanalytic – that would appear to respond to that question. Embodied simulation, most recently, has been expanded to include psychoanalysis. Defined by Gallese as "a neurofunctional mechanism enabling viewers to re-enact observed gestures, affects, and movements," this theoretical view, with its activation of a "non-representational, affective unconscious rooted in bodily memory and relational experience," is said to "participate in the ongoing formation of subjectivity," echoing the notion of the *becoming of mind* at the center of this book. Yet, while Gallese includes the unconscious in his increasingly psychoanalytically-informed view of aesthetic experience, the "reconceptualization of the unconscious" that he offers is that of a "*sensorimotor and affective unconscious*" which differs substantially from the classical perspective, the Freudian view grounded in the idea of repression.[72] It differs from the focus on the neurophysiology of the primary and secondary mentation essential to Freud's view of the mind, a view to which Friston subscribes and which is grounded in the notion of drive as originating in biological need. Whether conceived as culminating in pleasure (Freud) or satiation (as revised by Solms: "pleasure […] tells you that you are heading in the right *direction*, but it is not the *end* of a drive"[73]), *it is this force, this entropic momentum, which produces the play with the unreal, which induces the curiosity and creativity in which the aesthetic experience resides.* Unlike the "transitional, transformative engagement with the world" that Gallese defines (in accordance with Donald Winnicott and Ernst Kris) as the psychoanalytically comprehensible site of aesthetic experience, drive, as inherent in the aesthetic encounter, cannot be eliminated by the privileging of what Gallese views as "a pre-reflective, motorically grounded enactment of the movement encoded in the image." Even when temporally framed in terms of what Freud called *Nachträglichkeit* (or "deferred action"), meaning in art cannot be reductively defined as the reactivation of "previous embodied schemata – motor, affective, mnemonic – imbued with a new salience." Even when affectively framed in terms of the "resonance" reanimating "the viewer's affective unconscious," the artistic image cannot be reductively defined as "a *neuro-affective releaser*," however much of an expansion of embodied aesthetics Gallese now proposes.[74] No more instinctual than the development of empathy – the affective ground upon which embodied simulation, with its reliance on the theory of mirror neurons, has rested, but a developmental accomplishment achieved through the "continuities and discontinuities" to which both Neubauer, Abrams, and Balzert's prospective observational study and Solms' research and writings attest[75] – the memories and simulated movements produced by the visual encounter rely upon the *experiential acquisition* of meaningful associations. This is to recognize the pleasure-related, inspiration- and excitement-filled element inherent in their predictive (as opposed to corrective) capacity.

This is perhaps most easily appreciated in the relation of music to time: Entrainment (the synchronization of bodily movement with the audial perception of rhythmic pulsation) is how prediction, anticipation of the pulsations to come, occurs. Is the pleasure of such anticipation embedded in a counteractive or restorative function, in the minimization of the uncertain, or in the *prospect* of uncertainty minimization itself? Is the feel of the rhythm beholden to a cognitive apprehension of the temporal creation, a cortical recognition of the musical shaping of time, or to a self-propagating process of neural stimulation, a self-perpetuating neuronal activity known as "action potential" that stimulates the release of dopamine?

Attributing greater significance to the conceptual frame of a visual work of art than its aesthetic execution, Ladislav Kesner has noted with regard to "resistance and rejections" that "continue to be a fairly common reaction to much contemporary art" (but do they, one is inclined to ask?), with regard to "the failure of much contemporary art to incite any interest on the part of the audience" (but does it?), the lack of prediction error generation. For some, like Kesner, art that is "challenging," that is in some way difficult to relate to, "requires deliberate cognitive activity."[76] Others, like Floris P. de Lange et al., however, report that "Recent findings from both human neuroimaging and animal electrophysiology have revealed that prior expectations can modulate sensory processing at both early and late stages, and both before and after stimulus onset. The response modulation can take the form of either dampening the sensory representation or enhancing it via a process of sharpening."[77] The interplay between prediction and the actuality of sensory response, the neuromodulation that is an outcome of uncertainty, of predictive inaccuracy as it is of accuracy as well, cannot be denied. But, in the realm of the aesthetic, need the *correction* of such error be construed as the primary source of pleasure? Might not the *anticipation* itself be the source of the pleasure involved? Need the passing from greater uncertainty to lesser uncertainty alone, or even primarily, define the appreciation of a work of art? Need the resolution of prediction error provide the context for the subjective experience of art? Might not the paradigmatic shift in relation between emotion and cognition to which Seth and Friston, for example, attest – the paradigmatic shift from their dichotomization to their unification via the use of prediction as opposed to prediction error – provide a more legitimate platform from which to regard the *experience of*, which is to say the *subjective feeling* constituting the response to, the work of art? Or, to put it otherwise, is this not the curiosity and creativity of SEEKING impelled by the making of and the response to art?

Friston's "Law" or Beckett's "Mess"?

I.

"All the quantities in a self-organizing system that can change will change to minimize free energy."[78] This is what Solms, with only a glimmer of a chuckle, refers to as "Friston's Law." It is in accordance with this "law," with this theory of predictive processing, that we learn; it is in accordance with this "law" that "continuities" and "discontinuities" (to cite Neubauer, Abrams, and Balzert) occur. Predictions emanate from the model that generates the mind, the model that allows for the conceptualization of memories as "experiential priors," and the "forward pull" of development as of the life force itself. It is the temporality of prediction and the perpetual resolution of errors in expectation that take us far from the deterministic dichotomizing of nature and nurture, far from the falsity of that dichotomy – false insofar as during development of the brain genes and the environment work together[79] – and validate the "becoming mind" perspective with which I began this book.

Freud defined "drive" as "a measure of the demand made upon the mind for work in consequence of its connection with the body." It was in considering "the pressure" of a drive, the "force" of the phenomenon he located "on the frontier between the mental and the somatic," in "considering mental life from a *biological* point of view," that he laid the foundation for "Friston's Law."[80] In fact, it is the uniformity of Freud's view of consciousness, of primary and secondary process thinking, and much of what has emerged in recent years in neuroscience that has led not only to validation of the theory of predictive coding, but to the discipline of neuropsychoanalysis. And it is this discipline that addresses the interrelation, the interdependence even, of the neurophysiological and psychical substrates of both developmental and symptomatologic phenomena.

Extending beyond the ocular-centric frame of some and the embodied simulation frame of others – each leading to conclusions inherently problematic by virtue of *their omission of the dynamic reality at play, the omission of the affective constitution of subjectivity* – the neuropsychoanalytic perspective enriches understanding of aesthetic experience in fundamental ways. I will return to this in Chapter Five where the limits of psychobiography will be shown to compete in insufficiency with the conclusions drawn by some theoreticians of predictive coding as referred to already. For the moment, I wish to stress the importance of yet another "law" in such experience, what Solms terms the "Law of Affect."

As Solms describes it, affect is a fundamental means of ensuring homeostatic equilibrium. The foundation of consciousness (as we saw in Chapter One), it ensures learning and is the means by which one survives the unpredicted. In a word, it is "the biological function of experience."[81] "Artworks are … as dead as doornails,"[82] we recall once again Solms having proclaimed when writing of the absence of subjectivity in an object of perception such as the work of art. Indeed, one cannot empathize with artworks and the possibility of empathic error is therefore non-existent in aesthetics. "Artworks are … as dead as doornails," he declared, stressing the absence we take for granted but rarely see fit to articulate. In subjectivity, as noted earlier, Husserl, Sartre, and others more recently have sought the therapeutic solution to the illness of inhumanity. Today, Julia Kristeva, for one, fervently seeks in the subjectivity of the written word the potential for the kind of revolt needed to defy the crises of humanity. In art, as in psychoanalysis, she finds the antidote to determinism, the means of mutiny, the way toward freedom from the crises that have befallen us with autocracy, war, natural disaster, and illness throughout the world. How are we to understand that if the work of art, however much we speak of the intersubjectivity of author and reader, painter and viewer, is not a subjective entity? How are we to understand that abstract no less than figurative art bestows upon us the predictive functions ascribed to the brain that Friston and Solms, and Bayes before them, have established? How are we to understand that abstraction itself contains the pleasure assumed to be associated only with the however-much-delayed or absent recognition of the real?

"High solitary art uniquely self-pervaded, one with its wellhead in a hiddenmost of spirit, not to be clarified in any other light," wrote Beckett of the "strangeness" of Jack B. Yeats' art to which he paid homage. It is precisely the "strangeness," toward whose understanding "the sureties kindly unearthed in [the artist's] favour" offer "no great help," that affords instantaneous pleasure:

> In images of such breathless immediacy as these there is no occasion, no time given, no room left, for the lenitive of comment. None in this impetus of need that scatters them loose to the beyond of vision. None in this great inner real where phantoms quick and dead, nature and void, all that ever and that never will be, join in a single evidence for a single testimony. None in this final mastery which submits in trembling to the unmasterable.

And thus he concludes: "Merely bow in wonder."[83] While some place creative experience within the parameters of a cognitive mediation, what Beckett calls the "two great temptations, that of the real and that of the lie" – temptations that the Cubist painter Henry Hayden, for one, resisted, resulting for Beckett in the beauty of Hayden's work – emotional processes are clearly not to be forgotten.[84] Such is the awe the writer experienced before the "breathless immediacy" of Yeats' art.

Some, however, as it has been my objective to show, integrate the need to explore the source of such wonder by situating the drive that is curiosity and the neuronal circuitry subtending it within the frame of cognition and active knowing. Still others are increasingly questioning whether detection of the familiar and the diminution of uncertainty with which it is congruent are requisite to aesthetic appreciation or reward. Whether perceptual challenge or epistemological quest, abstraction clearly motivates interest in and appreciation of art. As Claudia Muth, Gesche Westphal-Fitch, and Claus-Christian Carbon have demonstrated, the triggering of interest (curiosity) and the fostering of subjective meaning (creativity) in the observer of an ambiguous visual artwork is an unquestionable source of aesthetic pleasure.[85] As Muth, Carbon, and Vera M. Hesslinger have also empirically shown, the greater the subjective perception of ambiguity, the greater the positive emotional response independent of any determination of beauty and of the solvability of ambiguous imagery. In fact, what they found to be at play in the appreciation of abstract artworks were personality factors relating not to ambiguity resolution, but ambiguity tolerance as well as the "*powerfulness of affect*," perceptual and cognitive alike.[86]

Ambiguous images often stimulate by way of their challenge greater curiosity and thereby appreciation. So, too, ambivalence, with its conflicting valences, has been shown to increase attention and heighten arousal increasing the potential for a positive response over time.[87] Beckett's writing is imbued with contradiction, ambivalence, opposition, and conflict, all expressing the impenetrable "opposition between art and life," as Carla Locatelli has termed it and which she explains as follows:

> Beckett no longer believed that the aim of the writer was to create images of life; in fact, he was opposed to the creation of "mimetic images," inasmuch as they do not reveal precisely the fact that they *are* images, and accurately conceal their figurative, conventional quality. He, on the contrary, wanted to

> create images of the "invisible images," so that he could constantly remind the reader that genres are essentially a convention, and literature a place where words "take their parts" before they actually relate to things.[88]

The idea of ridding literature of words, creating a "literature of the non-word," as Beckett described it in a 1937 letter as that to which he was aspiring, was elucidated by him as follows:

> It is indeed getting more and more difficult, even pointless, for me to write in formal English. And more and more my language appears to me like a veil which one has to tear apart in order to get to those things (or the nothingness) lying behind it. Grammar and style! To me they seem to have become as irrelevant as the Biedermeier bathing suit or the imperturbability of a gentleman. A mask. [...] To drill one hole after another into [language] until that which lurks behind, be it something or nothing, starts seeping through – I cannot imagine a higher goal for today's writer.
>
> Or is literature alone to be left behind on that old, foul road long ago abandoned my music and painting? Is there something paralyzingly sacred contained within the unnature of the word that does not belong to the elements of the other arts? Is there any reason why that terrifyingly arbitrary materiality of the word surface should not be dissolved, as for example the sound surface of Beethoven's Seventh Sympathy is devoured by huge black pauses, so that for pages on end we cannot perceive it other than a dizzying path of sounds connecting unfathomable chasms of silence?[89]

Relating to reality by way of the "non-word," by way of the dematerialization or dissolution of the "word surface": In what greater "mess," in what greater chaos, might one's aesthetic experience consist?

Writing of the Dutch painter Bram Van Velde's art education, critic Daniel Soutif once described how Van Velde "exchanged the knowledge he had acquired, and its promises, for the essential, the purely existential, dimension of painting."[90] Commenting on how this painter's gouaches, with "their lack of pigmentation boring holes of radical blankness in the image," echo Samuel Beckett's writing, on how their "sense of the arbitrariness, the existential contingency, of the very gesture of painting" resonates with Beckett's writing, Soutif observed the randomness, the unpredictability, the uncertainty inscribed within this visual artist's late work.[91] "Looking at his mature works," wrote Soutif, "one gets a feeling of ceaseless effort [...] to engender a necessity where none had existed before. Existence equals contingency, and contingency is perhaps more blatant within the limits of what is called painting than it is anywhere else. Why these forms? Why these colors? The naked surface on which they have come to dance, after all, wanted nothing, absolutely nothing."[92] Like others of their time, what preoccupied Van Velde and Beckett was a "total ontological engagement,"[93] as Soutif referred to it, whether a literary or visual "dialectic of the possible and the impossible, the expressible and the inexpressible, the visible and the invisible."[94] And therein the pleasure of the art was to be found:

> It is a strange pleasure, in the end, to paint as Van Velde did. It is a reciprocally strange pleasure to look at the result. For what is a pleasure that is nourished by the impossible [...]? Pleasures, nevertheless, exist here, and on every side. Van Velde's art is like a paradoxical dance that in spite of certain appearances is not the dance of death: it makes visual pleasure out of uncertainty and risk. That is why it is impossible to resist the fascination of the accidental forms, capsized colors, tentative transparencies, trickles, and spontaneous iridescences that make up this unparalleled painting. It was undoubtedly this fascination that led Van Velde to say, in an extraordinary, self-reflexive formula, that painting "is an eye, a blind eye, which sees what blinds it."[95]

Nothing could be further from the belief that the pleasure of art resides solely or even primarily in its minimization of uncertainty than this utterance of Van Velde himself: "Art is risk. What is the point of doing something that one is capable of doing?"[96] Or this "terrible critique [by Van Velde] of the too happily resolved painting of a colleague," as Soutif put it: "'It is a painting in which there was nothing to go wrong.'"[97]

If pleasure is to be found in the minimization of free energy, in the reduction of surprise and uncertainty, as Friston, Solms, and others have convincingly argued, are we really to assume that art which in some way reproduces reality while remaining of the imagination, while remaining in itself unreal, that art which is most like reality though not of it, art which is more realistic and representational while uniquely imaginative in its interpretive dimension, is of the highest order? Are we really to assume that art which seeks to deny replication is less valued, less prized for its casting off of the recognizable, the more easily known? As we have seen, some would say so. "Of all abstract art our theory predicts that we will be most impressed by paintings in which we can, with some labor, distinguish recognizable predictable forms," Van de Cruys and Wagemans have written.[98] And Kesner has situated what he calls "[t]he well-documented aversion to modern art" in the same framework while claiming that "once the minimization of prediction error at the level of object recognition concludes the viewing, there is no expectation of further reward and hence no motivation for a prolonged viewing and thinking about the work."[99]

Others would note, myself included, that, contrary to the above, from Picasso and Braque to Kandinsky and Dalí, from Rothko and Pollock to de Kooning and Franz Kline, modernist painting, like Beckett's unwording of literature, however glaring its abstraction from reality, has shown itself to be among the most highly valued forms of expression. The rejection of realism in favor of the abstract, generally speaking, or, more specifically, of any distinctly modernist movement, brought with it innovation and experimentation that made uncertainty, the unknowable, and surprisal their very *raisons d'être*. And the work of the great many artists seeking the least representational form of expression could hardly be more highly esteemed.

Does that contradict "Friston's Law"? Does it follow that because of our biologically determined need to minimize free energy, to do away with perceptual input that does not conform to expectation, to probability and prediction, abstract art would be, to whatever degree, inherently less acceptable than its representational counterpart? Minimizing free energy means minimizing surprise; minimizing surprise serves us physiologically. Indeed, "[p]erception," Solms explains, "is an endeavor to self-generate the incoming sensory signals and thereby explain them away." As he tells it, "Brain circuits literally *do* compute prior probability distributions and then send predictive messages to sensory neurons, in an endless effort to dampen incoming signals; and perception literally *does* involve comparisons between the predicted and actual distributions, resulting in computations of posterior probability. The resultant inferences are what perception *actually* is."[100] And thus the Bayesian brain (as noted in the previous chapter) is at the forefront of cognitive neuroscience today.

Yet, if the idea of an underappreciation of abstract art as outlined above is not tenable, if it is not valid despite the validity of "Friston's Law" and the "Bayesian brain," *why* is it not? The idea that advancing from more to less uncertainty is pleasurable is certainly justifiable both psychologically and biologically speaking. The idea that aesthetic experience is inherently negative or unpleasurable when content is unrecognizable is not. Why? Is it because we can tolerate, even take pleasure in, uncertainty when we anticipate the unpredictable, such as in a museum setting as Van de Cruys and Wagemans would have it? Or is it because, as they state, prediction errors are not acted upon in art as they are in real life?[101] Many are those who found in the non-referential the means to move away from the barbarity of World War II. Abstraction offered harmony, silence even, where chaos, uncertainty, and the senseless reigned. And abstraction, then as before and after as well, offered something more: A something that is nothing at all. Perhaps, then, it is because "Art is nothing. A little bit of nothing."[102] And in the perception of that nothingness there is an investment of affect just as there is in conscious awareness.

II.

In 1980, French philosopher Christian Delacampagne remarked, "What is new is not that we are in a crisis; it is that the crisis is unnamable. It is that there no longer exists a conceptual network, a grid, science or ideology that would allow for thinking, simply, of crisis."[103] Friston's formulations of the Free Energy Principle, of learning formulated in accordance with this theory, allows us to do just that, for *crisis* – understood not in the sense of catastrophe from which it was differentiated earlier and not in the sense of calamity in the colloquial sense – *is precisely what occurs in the absence of learning.* According to Delacampagne, long ago "any connection with the various traditions that allowed [...] for formulation – and thereby assumption – of the crisis" was destroyed:

> We killed all speech of which we were the sons. Since then, we have been orphans. Orphans who question themselves, more than ever, about their origins...
>
> Consequently, I will not try to imagine a new theory of crisis – to be added to the procession of those we already have [...].
>
> Rather, I will force myself to say how I hope, not to leave the crisis, but instead to set myself within it.
>
> Joyfully, if possible.[104]

"Joyfully"? How might that be? How might one set oneself *within crisis and derive pleasure* if pleasure ensues from the minimization of uncertainty, from the minimization of prediction error and of unexpected surprise to which Van de Cuys, Kesner, and others inspired by Friston's free energy theory have directed our attention? How might one set oneself *within crisis and derive pleasure* if crisis in accordance with this theory is defined as the very state of unpleasure ensuing from uncertainty?

How might Freud's idea that pleasure and unpleasure are a function of alterations in the strength of the stimulus relate to the pleasure of aesthetic experience? To understand this apparent contradiction in the context of aesthetic experience I turn to the following by Jacques Garelli:

> Il y a un paradoxe de l'activité poétique qui est la mesure de sa condition. Ouverture sur le monde, le poème est, dans l'acte du dévoilement, cela même qui est dévoilé. Regard, il se fait voir. Lumière, il s'éclaire. Révélateur, il ne révèle qu'en étant lui-même révélé.
>
> (There is a paradox of poetic activity that is the measure of its condition. Opening onto the world, the poem is, in the act of unveiling, that which is unveiled. A gaze, it makes itself seen. Light, it illuminates itself. Revealer, it reveals only in being itself revealed.)

It is in "the structure of this ambiguity" that the poetic or any other kind of art "rend présent ce qui ouvre une présence" ("renders present that which opens a presence").[105] In other words, Friston's notion of crisis and the pleasure that follows escaping the uncertainty of surprise is both the antithesis of poetic activity as described by Garelli and not, once one considers the paradox he puts forth. For there is pleasure not only in the diminution of surprise, in the certainty that accompanies recognition, but in the realization of the art work as revelatory both of what it makes seen and of itself as a process of revelation.

Beckett took this paradox a step farther when, writing of modern painting, he declared that "L'objet de la représentation résiste toujours à la représentation" ("The object of representation always resists representation").[106] He said the same of literary art: "chaque fois qu'on veut faire faire aux mots un véritable travail de transbordement, chaque fois qu'on veut leur faire exprimer autre chose que des mots, ils s'alignent de façon à s'annuler mutuellement" ("every time that one wants to make of words a veritable work of transshipment, every time that one wants to make them express something other than words, they align in such a way as to mutually annul each other").[107] And it was this belief in art as *fundamentally untranslatable of the world outside it*, this belief in the *unrepresentability of the object*, that was the basis of his plays and fiction. If his effort was to depict anything in his art, it was what Garelli called "l'immanence de l'être" ("the immanence of being"),[108] what Beckett called "the mess": "One cannot speak anymore of being, one must speak only of the mess. When Heidegger and Sartre speak of a contrast between being and existence, they may be right, I don't know, but their language is too philosophical for me. I am not a philosopher. One can only speak of what is in front of him, and that now is simply the mess."[109] As the writer's aptly named character the Unnamable says in the novel of the same name: "People with things, people without things, things without people, what does it matter, I flatter myself it will not take me long to scatter them, whenever I choose, to the winds."[110] Unable to be articulated *as he is*, the Unnamable forsakes his multiple individualities in resigned acceptance of the annihilation this indetermination implies: "Nothing to do but stretch out comfortably on the rack, in the blissful knowledge you are nobody for all eternity."[111] As previously noted, it is *Breath*, with its thirty-five-second interplay of light, the cry of a newborn, and recorded breath, that offers the most dramatic example of a non-linguistic, metaphorically visual and oral enactment of life experience. So condensed is the event that any portrayal of character, to say nothing of speech, is excluded and the play is but a theatricalization of the playwright's existential vision itself.

As I have discussed at length elsewhere,[112] Beckett writes, in an essay on the brothers Geer and Bram van Velde, that in the economy of art what is not said is the light of what is said and that every presence is absence. In a second such essay he more closely targets the dialectic as process: painting as an endless unveiling of the unavailable, a seeing of what cannot be seen. In both essays, the contradiction inherent in creative expression, the visible rendering of what cannot be seen, is shown to stem not from a conflict of semiotic origin, from the incongruity of sign and what it designates, but from the transparency and opacity of the world itself. It is precisely in their projection of this paradigm, of the world as phenomenon of disclosure and resistance at once, that these essays reveal the author's anaesthetic orientation to visual art, an orientation comparable to the parity of Beckett's own theatre art with lived space and time, what critic Ruby Cohn famously referred to as "theatereality." Ultimately, Beckett will more fully develop the contradiction that the ontological and even inherently interrogative nature of art present, but the point is that, as he explains it, painting is an accommodation of the inexplicable "mess" or chaos of existence.

Like Martin Heidegger's phenomenology of art, Beckett's thinking about painting, reminiscent of the philosopher's in "The Origin of the Work of Art," transcends aesthetic valorization in representation to resituate it in revelation. Heidegger's focus is the work at work, the unveiling of a thing in truth. Beckett similarly situates art on the level of the primordial apprehension of the real.[113] Insofar as art fails for the impossibility of reproduction, not only is its failure not its end, but art is said to originate precisely therein: "Ever tried. Ever failed. No matter. Try again. Fail again. Fail better." These were the words he wrote in his 1983 novella *Worstward Ho*. It is by its very failure to represent that art is authentically innovative and the artist truly creative. And it is therein that the "joyful," the pleasure, is found.

"L'art," as the late philosopher Henri Maldiney expressed it, "est la vérité du sensible" ("Art is the truth of feeling").[114] Understood as illustrative, understood in the imitative realm of signaling something other than itself, the work of art held no more aesthetic value for Maldiney than for Beckett, just as it held no more such value for Beckett than for Garelli or for others influenced by Heidegger and, even more so, by Merleau-Ponty. Rather, the artwork was seen as dependent only upon its own rhythmic (which is to say spatiotemporal) emergence, and therefore as perpetually in-formation. I will return to the notion of form as distinguished from image in Chapter Four where I will explore the notion of what I term the "imageless image." *My point here, however, concerns the active mode, the generativity, the affective energy through which the work of art reveals itself as actualization as opposed to illustration or representation. For it is therein that aesthetic experience may truly be said to reside.*

As we saw earlier, the neurobiological significance of creativity lies in its goal-oriented, motivational predisposition toward the satisfaction of curiosity, the questioner's "need" to know. Whatever the verbal or visual image produced, however many times the image destroyed and remade, rather than as a re-presentation of an external reality, the neurophilosophical perspective, like the metaneuropsychological, allows for its understanding as a response to endogenous demands. This is not to say, of course, that the work of art is not a manifestation of unconscious wishes. In "Creative Writers and Day-Dreaming," Freud articulates the relation between fantasy/dream and literary creativity precisely in the context of unconscious wish-fulfillment. The wish traverses the past, present, and future by way of memory, present provocation, and gratification in the creative work. And this is precisely where Solms' revision of Freud's *Project* takes us to the heart of the matter: What Solms offers is an understanding of *why*. What is the "meta*neuro*psychological" *raison d'être* of that novel or poem, of that painting? That is the question at hand. Not, is it good or bad, poorly written or beautifully painted? Such, of course, is the realm of literary or art criticism. Rather, more to the point, *why* did it come to be? What motivational purpose was served? The answer lies not within the reductionism of psychobiography, a practice grounded in supposition and relegated to the surface of understanding.

Sontag said it best when she wrote, "[I]nterpretation is the revenge of the intellect upon art. Even more. It is the revenge of the intellect upon the world."[115] At issue, as Sontag articulated in her masterful essay "Against Interpretation," is not content, but *purpose: the endogenous, fundamentally affective, and self-organizing objective of self-preservation achieved through the prediction of outcome.* What Solms puts in high relief is the legitimacy of James Joyce's declaration: "A man of genius [by which is meant, in *Ulysses*, the artist] makes no mistakes. His errors are volitional and are the portals of discovery."[116] Otherwise written, "Artists make no mistakes. Their errors are homeostatically invaluable and are the predictive portals of discovery that are fundamentally disambiguating." And yet…

One's identification with characters, their experiences and feelings, whether understood as empathic, enactivist, or more purely reflective, is often the focus of interpretation, particularly psychoanalytic, on the "tacit assumption," Pinchas Noy and Dorit Noy-Sharav have written, "that meanings are related to a narrative, and the function of interpretation is therefore to the hidden narrative line out of unconscious symbolizations, condensations and other distortions." However true that may be, as they further note, "The problem is that such an approach is justified only in the case of interpreting content, but not for interpreting form."[117] Indeed, what is to be said of the response to art, whatever the genre, that is so abstract as to be without content as such? This is the "mess" that Beckett brings to the fore: the "terrible materiality of the word surface" he sought to expose, the "literature of the unword" he sought to create.

If empathy as the result of embodied simulation, of the identification with the other by way of experiencing with them or inferring from them, cannot occur to the extent that there is no other, how we explain our appreciation, or lack thereof, of the aesthetic object has been the focus of this chapter. In the chapter that follows, the lack of a subject impeding empathic resonance will give way to the lack of something assumed to be at least as fundamental in visual art: the image. In turning from the subjectless subject to the imageless image and concluding my dispute with those in cognitive neuroscience who, in their application of the Free Energy Principle to art, deduce, above all else, that the pleasure of art resides in recognition, I am reminded of Beckett's aptly worded declaration: "The danger is in the neatness of identifications."[118]

Notes

1 Mark Solms, "Empathy as Developmental Achievement: Beyond Embodied Simulation," *Neuroscience and Critique: Exploring the Limits of the Neurological Turn*, ed. Jan De Vos and Ed Pluth (Routledge, 2016), 205.

2 Gilbert Simondon, *Individuation in Light of Notions of Form and Information*, trans. Taylor Adkins (University of Minnesota Press, 2005/2020), 363 (emphasis added).

3 Mark Solms, "The Hard Problem of Consciousness and the Free Energy Principle," *Frontiers in Psychology* 9, article 2714 (2019): 7.
4 Mark Solms, *The Hidden Spring: A Journey to the Source of Consciousness* (W.W. Norton, 2021), 236.
5 Robert Pepperell, "Being Alive to the World: An Artist's Perspective on Predictive Processing," *Philosophical Transactions of the Royal Society*, 2023, B379:20220429. doi:10.1098/rstb.2022.0429
6 Sander Van de Cruys and Johan Wagemans, "Putting Reward in Art: A Tentative Error Account of Visual Art," *I-Perception* 2 (2011): 1035.
7 Van de Cruys and Wagemans, "Putting Reward in Art," 1036.
8 Van de Cruys and Wagemans, "Putting Reward in Art," 1037.
9 Van de Cruys and Wagemans, "Putting Reward in Art," 1040, 1041.
10 Van de Cruys and Wagemans, "Putting Reward in Art," 1048–49.
11 Van de Cruys and Wagemans, "Putting Reward in Art," 1052.
12 Sander Van de Cruys, Jo Bervoets, and Agnes Moors, "Preferences Need Inferences: Learning, Valuation, and Curiosity in Aesthetic Experience," in *The Routledge International Handbook of Neuroaesthetics*, ed. Martin Skov and Marcos Nadal (Routledge, 2023), 494.
13 Mary Ann Caws, *Symbolism, Dada, Surrealisms* (Reaktion Books, 2024), 121.
14 Caws, *Symbolism, Dada, Surrealisms*, 15.
15 Joyce Cary, *Art and Reality: Ways of Creative Process* (Harper & Brothers, 1958), 72.
16 Donald Judd, "New York: The Art World," in *Arts Yearbook 7* (The Art Digest Inc., 1964), 28.
17 Hilton Kramer, "Notes on Painting in New York," *Arts Yearbook 7* (The Art Digest Inc., 1964), 10, 20.
18 See Ladislav Kesner, "A Hole in a Piece of Cardboard and Predictive Brain: The Incomprehension of Modern Art in the Light of the Predictive Coding Paradigm," *Philosophical Transactions of the Royal Society*, B 379: 20220417. doi:10.1098/rstb.2022.0417
19 Kesner, "A Hole in a Piece of Cardboard and Predictive Brain."
20 Mario Livio, *Why? What Makes Us Curious?* (Simon & Schuster, 2017), 33.
21 Sigmund Freud, "Three Essays on Sexuality," *Standard Edition*, vol. 7, 178.
22 Van de Cruys, Bervoets and Moors, "Preferences Need Inferences," 493.
23 Mark Solms, "Revision of Drive Theory," *JAPA* 69, no. 6 (2022): 1067.
24 W.H. Auden, *Van Gogh: A Self-Portrait; Letters Revealing His Life as a Painter* (New York Graphic Society, 1961), 192.
25 Samuel Beckett, "Intercessions by Denis Devlin," in *Disjecta*, ed. Ruby Cohn (Grove Press, 1984), 91.
26 Lisa Feldman Barrett, "Knowledge vs. Creativity." https://iai.tv/video/knowledge-v-creativity?utm_source=YouTube&utm_medium=description
27 Merleau-Ponty, "Cézanne's Doubt" (1945), in *The Merleau-Ponty Aesthetics Reader: Philosophy and Painting*, ed. Galen A. Johnson (Northwestern University Press, 1993), 69. See also Evelyne Grossman, *La créativité de la crise* (Les Éditions de Minuit, 2020).
28 Grossman, *La créativité de la crise*, 82–83 (trans. mine).
29 See "Yo Yo Ma and the Meaning of Life," interview with David Marchese, *The New York Times Magazine*, Nov. 20, 2020.
30 See Jaak Panksepp and Colwyn Trevarthen, "The Neuroscience of Emotion in Music," in Stephen Malloch and Colwyn Trevarthen (eds.), *Communicative Musicality: Exploring the Basis of Human Companionship* (Oxford University Press, 2009), 105–46.

31 See Robert J. Zatorre, and Valorie N. Salimpoor, "Why Music Makes Our Brain Sing." *The New York Times* (June 7, 2013).
32 Edward Vessel, Gabrielle Starr, and Nava Rubin, "Art Reaches Within: Aesthetic Experience, the Self and the Default Mode Network," *Frontiers in Neuroscience* (2013), 6. https://doi.org/10.3389/fnins.2013.00258
33 Vessel, Starr, and Rubin, "Art Reaches Within," 7.
34 Vessel, Starr, and Rubin, "Art Reaches Within," 7.
35 Solms, "Revision of Drive Theory," 1052.
36 Qtd. by Eric R. Kandel in *Reductionism in Art and Brain Science* (Columbia University Press, 2016), 130.
37 Samuel Beckett, "Dante ... Bruno. Vico. Joyce," in *Disjecta*, ed. Ruby Cohn (Grove Press, 1984), 27.
38 Vittorio Gallese, "The Embodiment of Images: A View from the Brain-Body," paper presented at Psychoanalytic Dialogues conference, Rome, January 25, 2025.
39 Shaun Gallagher, "Empathy, Simulation, and Narrative," *Science in Context* 25, no. 3 (2012): 355.
40 David Freedberg and Vittorio Gallese, "Motion, Emotion and Empathy in Esthetic Experience," *TRENDS in Cognitive Sciences* 11, no. 5 (2007). doi: 10.1016/j.tics.2007.02.0
41 See, for example, Vittorio Gallese and George Lakoff, "The Brain's Concepts: The Role of the Sensory-Motor System in Conceptual Knowledge," *Cognitive Neuropsychology* 22, no. 3–4 (2005): 455–79. doi:10.1080/02643290442000310
42 Freedberg and Gallese, "Motion, Emotion and Empathy in Esthetic Experience."
43 Merleau-Ponty, "Cézanne's Doubt," 65.
44 G.A. Johnson, "Ontology and Painting: 'Eye and Mind,'" in *The Merleau-Ponty Aesthetics Reader: Philosophy and Painting*, ed. Galen A. Johnson (Northwestern University Press, 1993), 49.
45 Johnson, "Ontology and Painting: 'Eye and Mind,'" 48.
46 Merleau-Ponty, "Cézanne's Doubt," 65.
47 Merleau-Ponty, "Eye and Mind" (1961), in *The Merleau-Ponty Aesthetics Reader: Philosophy and Painting*, ed. Galen A. Johnson (Northwestern University Press, 1993), 127.
48 Merleau-Ponty, "Eye and Mind," 128.
49 Merleau-Ponty, "Eye and Mind," 127 (emphasis added).
50 Johnson, "Ontology and Painting: 'Eye and Mind,'" 48.
51 Merleau-Ponty, "Eye and Mind," 123.
52 Merleau-Ponty, "Cézanne's Doubt" 63 (emphasis added).
53 Merleau-Ponty, "Cézanne's Doubt," 63.
54 Merleau-Ponty, "Cézanne's Doubt," 63 (emphasis added).
55 Merleau-Ponty, "Cézanne's Doubt," 69.
56 Merleau-Ponty, "Cézanne's Doubt," 64.
57 Merleau-Ponty, "Cézanne's Doubt," 63–64 (emphasis added).
58 Merleau-Ponty, "Eye and Mind," 129.
59 Merleau-Ponty, "Cézanne's Doubt," 67.
60 Samuel Beckett, *Breath* (1969), in *The Collected Shorter Plays of Samuel Beckett* (Grove Press, 1984), 211.
61 Cf. Sozita Goudouna, *Beckett's Breath: Anti-theatricality and the Visual Arts* (Edinburgh University Press, 2018), 124.
62 Laura Salisbury, "'What Is the Word': Beckett's Aphasic Modernism," *Journal of Beckett Studies* 17, no. 1–2 (2009): 78–126. doi:10.3366/E0309520709000090
63 For more on this distinction, see Goudouna, *Beckett's Breath: Anti-theatricality and the Visual Arts*, 125.

64 Samuel Beckett, *Not I* (1972), in *The Collected Shorter Plays of Samuel Beckett* (Grove Press, 1984), 215.
65 Samuel Beckett, *What Where*, in *The Collected Shorter Plays of Samuel Beckett* (Grove Press, 1984), 316.
66 Martin Esslin, *The Theatre of the Absurd* (Anchor Books, 1961), 46.
67 Pepperell, "Being Alive to the World."
68 Clement Greenberg, "The Crisis of the Easel Picture," in *Clement Greenberg: Art and Culture* (Beacon Press, 1961; first published in *Partisan Review*, April 1948), 157.
69 Anil K. Seth, "Interoceptive Inference, Emotion, and the Embodied Self," *Trends in Cognitive Sciences* 17, no. 11 (2013): 571.
70 Anil K. Seth and Karl Friston, "Active Interoceptive Inference and the Emotional Brain," *Philosophical Transactions of the Royal Society*, 2016. B37120160007. doi:10.1098/rstb.2016.0007
71 Claudia Muth et al., "Expecting the Unexpected: How Gallery Visitors Experience Semantic Instability in Art," *Art & Perception* 5 (2017): 124–25.
72 Vittorio Gallese, "Aesthetics and the Unconscious: Toward an Embodied Neuroscience of the Image," JAPA, December 4, 2025. DOI: 10.1177/00030651251394305.
73 Solms, "Revision of Drive Theory," 1053.
74 Gallese, "Aesthetics and the Unconscious."
75 See, in particular, Solms, "Revision of Drive Theory," 1079, note 37.
76 Kesner, "A Hole in a Piece of Cardboard and Predictive Brain."
77 Floris P. de Lange, Micha Heilbron, and Peter Kok, "How Do Expectations Shape Perception?" *Trends in Cognitive Sciences* 22, no. 9 (2018): 764–79.
78 Solms, *The Hidden Spring*, 177.
79 Cf. Cristina Alberini, "Early Life Learning and the Biological Basis of Individuality," lecture presented at the 24th International Neuropsychoanalysis Congress. Mt. Sinai School of Medicine, June 21, 2025.
80 Sigmund Freud, "Instincts and Their Vicissitudes," *Standard Edition*, vol. 14, 122, 121. It should be noted that *Trieb*, as it appears in Freud's original German, was translated by James Strachey in the Standard Edition as "instinct" and by Solms in the *Revised Standard Edition* as "drive."
81 Solms, *The Hidden Spring*, 303.
82 Solms, "Empathy as Developmental Achievement," 205.
83 Samuel Beckett, "Homage to Jack B. Yeats," in *Disjecta*, ed. Ruby Cohn (Grove Press, 1984), 149.
84 Samuel Beckett, "Henri Hayden," in *Disjecta*, ed. Ruby Cohn (Grove Press, 1984), 150.
85 See Claudia Muth, Gesche Westphal-Fitch, and Claus-Christian Carbon, "Seeking (Dis)order: Ordering Appeals but Slight Disorder and Complex Order Trigger Interest," *Psychology of Aesthetics, Creativity, and the Arts* 15, no. 3 (2021): 439–57. doi:10.1037/aca0000284
86 Claudia Muth, Vera M. Hesslinger, and Claus-Christian Carbon, "The Appeal of Challenge in the Perception of Art: How Ambiguity, Solvability of Ambiguity, and the Opportunity for Insight Affect Appreciation," *Psychology of Aesthetics, Creativity, and the Arts* 9, no. 3 (2015): 206–16. doi:10.1037/a0038814
87 Claudia Muth and Claus-Christian Carbon, "Ambivalence of Artistic Photographs Stimulates Interest and the Motivation to Engage," *Psychology of Aesthetics, Creativity, and the Arts* 18, no. 3 (2024): 287–302. doi:10.1037/aca0000448
88 Carla Locatelli, *Unwording the World* (University of Pennsylvania Press, 1990), 55.

89 Samuel Beckett, "Letter to Axel Kaun" (July 9, 1937). *The Letters of Samuel Beckett 1929–1940*, ed. Martha Dow Fehsenfeld and Lois More Overbeck (Cambridge University Press, 2009), 518–19.
90 Daniel Soutif, "Flight into Whiteness: Bram Van Velde," in *Art Forum* (Summer 1990): 150.
91 Soutif, "Flight into Whiteness: Bram Van Velde," 151.
92 Soutif, "Flight into Whiteness: Bram Van Velde," 150–151.
93 Soutif, "Flight into Whiteness: Bram Van Velde," 152.
94 Soutif, "Flight into Whiteness: Bram Van Velde," 153.
95 Soutif, "Flight into Whiteness: Bram Van Velde," 153.
96 Soutif, "Flight into Whiteness: Bram Van Velde," 150.
97 Jacques Putman and Charles Juliet, *Bram van Velde* (Maeght, 1975), cited by Soutif, "Flight into Whiteness: Bram Van Velde," 150.
98 Van de Cruys and Wagemans, "Putting Reward in Art," 1052.
99 Ladislav Kesner, "The Predictive Mind and the Experience of the Visual Art Work," *Frontiers in Psychology* 5 (2014): 7.
100 Solms, *The Hidden Spring*, 176.
101 Van de Cruys and Wagemans, "Putting Reward in Art," 1041.
102 Selden Rodman, *Conversations with Artists 1909–2002* (The Delvin-Adair Co., 1957), 120.
103 Christian Delacampagne "Ce qu'Occident veut dire," *Le Débat*, no. 4 (September 1980): 19.
104 Delacampagne "Ce qu'Occident veut dire," 19.
105 Jacques Garelli, *La gravitation poétique* (Mercure de France, 1966), 9 (trans. mine).
106 Samuel Beckett, "Les peintres de l'empêchement," in *Disjecta*, ed. Ruby Cohn (Grove Press, 1984), 135 (trans. mine).
107 Samuel Beckett, "La peinture des van Velde ou le Monde et le Pantalon," in *Disjecta*, ed. Ruby Cohn (Grove Press, 1984), 125 (trans. mine).
108 Garelli, *La gravitation poétique*, 66.
109 Samuel Beckett to Tom F. Driver, Summer 1961, qtd. by Lawrence Graver and Raymond Federman, *The Critical Heritage* (Routledge, 1979), 219.
110 Samuel Beckett, *The Unnamable* (Grove Press, 1958), 4–5.
111 Beckett, *The Unnamable*, 71.
112 See Lois Oppenheim, *The Painted Word: Samuel Beckett's Dialogue with Art* (The University of Michigan Press, 2000), 77.
113 Oppenheim, *The Painted Word*, 77–78.
114 Henri Maldiney, *Regard, Parole, Espace* (L'âge d'homme, 1973), 153 (trans. mine).
115 Susan Sontag, *Against Interpretation* (Farrar, Straus and Giroux, 1961), 7.
116 James Joyce, *Ulysses* (Shakespeare and Company, 1922), 9.228–29.
117 Pinchas Noy and Dorit Noy-Sharav. "Art and Emotions," *International Journal of Applied Psychoanalytic Studies* 10, no. 2 (2013): 100.
118 Beckett, "Dante … Bruno. Vico. Joyce," 19.

Chapter 4

The "Imageless Image"

When the art editor of *The New York Times* wrote in 1943 of his bewilderment before the abstract paintings exhibited at the Wildenstein Gallery's show of fifty-five members of the Federation of Modern Painters & Sculptors, Adolph Gottlieb and Mark Rothko replied with a letter. Regarding a painting by Gottlieb, they wrote: "It is an easy matter to explain to the befuddled that 'The Rape of Persephone' is a poetic expression of the essence of the myth; the presentation of the concept of seed and its earth with all its brutal implications; the impact of elemental truth. Would you have us present this abstract concept with all its complicated feelings by means of a boy and girl lightly tripping?" And referring to a work by Rothko, "It is just as easy to explain 'The Syrian Bull', as a new interpretation of an archaic image, involving unprecedented distortions. Since art is timeless, the significant rendition of a symbol, no matter how archaic, has as full validity today as the archaic symbol had then. Or is the one 3000 years old truer?" "But these easy program notes can help only the simple-minded," Gottlieb and Rothko continued. "No possible set of notes can explain our paintings. Their explanation must come out of a consummated experience between picture and onlooker. The appreciation of art is a true marriage of minds." Insofar as it is the "communicative power" of the painting that constitutes for these Abstract *Expressionists* (note emphasis) its essential aesthetic value, their purpose was neither to defend nor enlighten for it was the work itself that was to demonstrate their aesthetic convictions.[1]

The Aesthetic Encounter

Meaning, construed as it is by contextualization, affective and cognitive alike, refers to what is in some way implicitly conveyed or explicitly expressed and consciously or unconsciously construed. Both the emergence of mind from its biological origin and the maturation of an individual's sense of self by way of memory and learning are instrumental in meaning making, the foundation of subjective experience. It is subjective experience that takes us from the dichotomy of wish-fulfillment and sublimation as inherent within a psychoanalytic perspective, on the one hand, and embodiment and neuronal arousal, on the

DOI: 10.4324/9781003566755-5

other, to psychoaesthetics and neuroaesthetics and to the unifying notion of what is limited neither to an affective nor a cognitive relation of the spectator or reader to visual, performative, or literary art. The components of aesthetic creation and reception are indivisible when one considers the energic generativity, the experiential evidence – whether understood as predictive and dependent upon an associative prototype or as something more direct and affectively resonant – intrinsic within the valorization of art. This is to say that it is in the context of an integration of the neural with the affective, the sensorial and dopaminergic with the emotional – in the context of the interdependence of brain with mind – that aesthetic experience is to be considered. Is it also to say that the prediction (or the inference in which it is grounded) reducing the uncertainty associated with free energy is irrelevant to the appreciation of art? Certainly not, even if a number of the conclusions reached by some adherents to the adaptation of the Free Energy Principle to aesthetic experience are not shared by all (myself included).

Indeed, to the extent that "becoming" – the persistent refrain of this book serving as a reminder that an individual is never simply who they are but who they perpetually are emerging to be – is a function of memory and learning, predictive coding has much to teach us with regard not only to everyday living, but to aesthetic experience as well. *How* we view a painting or sculpture, listen to music, read a literary text, or watch a performance at any given moment in time, *why* we are curious about this "object" that is but is not one and that morphs in conjunction with our subjective apprehension of it, and *what* accounts for its hedonic value are in some measure a function of the persistent generating and updating of our internal representations. Such mental representations predict perceptual feedback regarding aspects of the environment that is then matched with the actuality of perception. Though derived primarily from the concept of the German physicist Hermann von Helmholtz known as "unconscious inference" and, as already noted, that of Thomas Bayes known as "Bayes theorem," the theory of predictive coding has gained considerable traction only in recent years. It has, in fact, gained significant momentum of late in several disciplines, dramatically advancing our understanding of the functioning of the psyche in accordance with neuronal imperatives in aesthetic as well as scientific domains. Infiltrating the study of aesthetic experience, it is beginning to account for how various forms of art affect, in addition to the creator of the artwork, the viewer, listener, or reader.

Consider for a moment the pleasure of music. The neurotransmitter dopamine is released in the basal ganglia, the clusters of brain cells located below the cerebral cortex and over the mid-brain, in moments of pleasurable feeling. As the research team of Robert Zatorre and Valorie Salimpoor found, this reward system is activated in the moments of greatest emotional intensity of music listening, but not only in such moments: Some seconds before this activation phase, there is an anticipatory phase, a prediction of a sought-after effect.[2] But it is not only the chemical reaction that accounts for the pleasure involved. Research has additionally found that there is activation of the auditory cortex when music is imagined. As Zatorre and Salimpoor have noted, when one imagines the opening notes of Beethoven's Fifth Symphony, the cortex is highly stimulated. And it this capacity to hear music when one is not actually hearing it that allows for the creation of new musical arrangements as well as the reimagining of a musical work played in accordance with a different rhythm or other instruments.[3] Prediction, in a word, has much to do with creativity.

And, as we saw earlier, the neurobiological significance of creativity also lies in its goal-oriented, motivational predisposition toward the satisfaction of curiosity, the seeker's "need" to know. Whatever the mental representation, whatever the internal image produced, however many times it may be remade, the theory of predictive coding allows for its understanding as a response to endogenous demands. So, too, the production of the artwork and the listener, reader, or spectator's experience of it, each driven by knowledge, expectation, and curiosity as well.

Such responsiveness, it might also be noted, is not limited to a single aesthetic realm in a viewer's engagement with a particular work of art. One may hear music and feel like moving in conjunction with that rhythm. In addition to or instead of an inclination to so move, to move in accordance with the

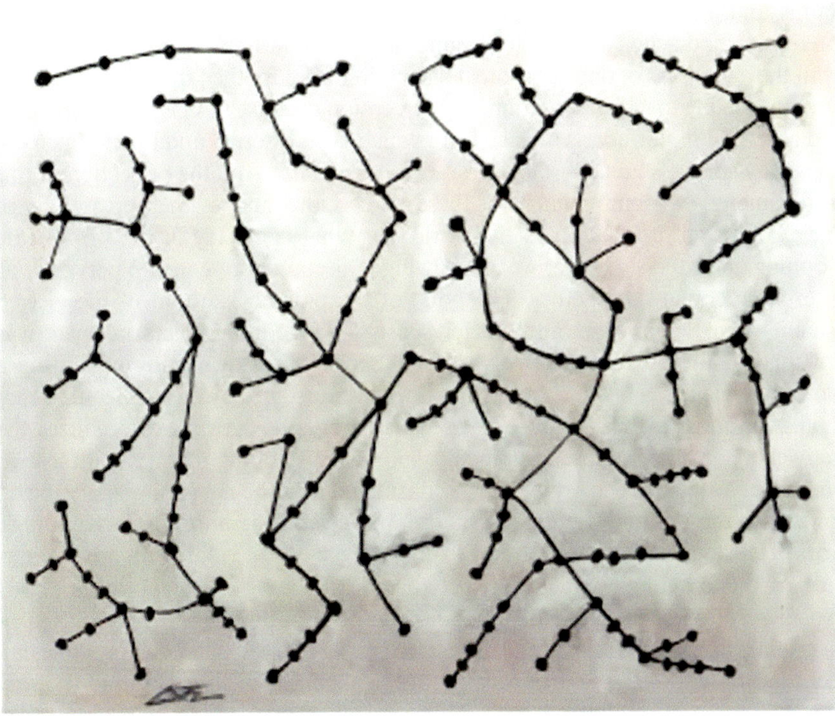

Figure 4.1 Untitled (Constellations) © 2024 The Estate of David Smith / Licensed by VAGA at Artists Rights Society (ARS), NY. Date: 1963 RoGallery.com, Long Island City, NY

rhythm aurally perceived, one may mentally envision choreography emanating not from a rhythm, not neuromuscularly, but pictorially. Conversely, one may see a visual artwork and feel a rhythm emanating from within it. This painting by David Smith is a case in point.

How are we to understand our experience of such a painting? Let us consider for a moment the perspective put forth by Gallese. Embodied simulation stresses the activation of the body as the principal means of aesthetic engagement. Structured affectively and temporally as well, in as much as bodily activation involves an arrestation and transformation of the perception of the image, it involves a reactivation of what Gallese refers to as "previous embodied schemata–motor, affective, mnemonic." In including the generation of "*sensorimotor anticipation*," it draws affect (and thereby empathy) into the experience to become both intercorporeal and relational, psychoanalytically speaking, or so Gallese reasons.[4] In the post-1940 paintings of Willem de Kooning, in whose work there may or may not be perceivable body imagery, there is what has been termed "a felt sense of space" which serves to ground one, so to speak, "in the world and history (in a physical sense)," as noted by art historian Valerie Hellstein.[5] The body, whether represented, suggested, or absent, is indeed fundamental to Abstract Expressionism, Hellstein claims, and, I would add, to all art. When Freud wrote of the ego's being "first and foremost a body-ego," he was suggesting not only that one's sense of self evolves from the awareness of one's corporeal distinction from mother, the giver of life, but from the feeling to which sensation and perception give rise: "A person's own body, and above all its surface, is a place from which both external and internal perceptions may spring," Freud wrote in *The Ego and the Id*.[6] And the projection of this embodiment – the embodiment of these perceptions and of the perceptions of one's bodily self in relation to the world – is what is at play in the work of de Kooning and others whether we are viewing it as content or color so pervasive as to exclude content altogether. The body of the painter, like that of the viewer, inhabits a particular space and this felt sense of de Kooning's pictorial space was not merely illusionistic but involved a felt sense of his own body inhabiting a particular place. "Since the ego is first and foremost a body ego – meaning that representations of the bodily self are at its core – the artwork externalizes the body ego," as Gilbert Rose explained.[7] And it is in so doing that it manifests two phenomena: the drive energy already considered and the rhythmic regulation so evident in the painting by David Smith.[8] In her consideration of de Kooning's work, Hellstein signals, moreover, the importance of "the materiality of the surface of the painting": "It is not just that de Kooning was painting sexually explicit, erotic images of women, but also that the surfaces of his paintings 'feel' a certain way. […] The surface of *Women Singing II* is slick and creamy. One can feel the twisting of the figures because of the slickness of the paint and the way they feel in their shallow space."[9] This kind of resonance has been admirably discussed by Gallese and others to demonstrate that one sensorially feels one's way into the art to experience the multiple dimensions at play.

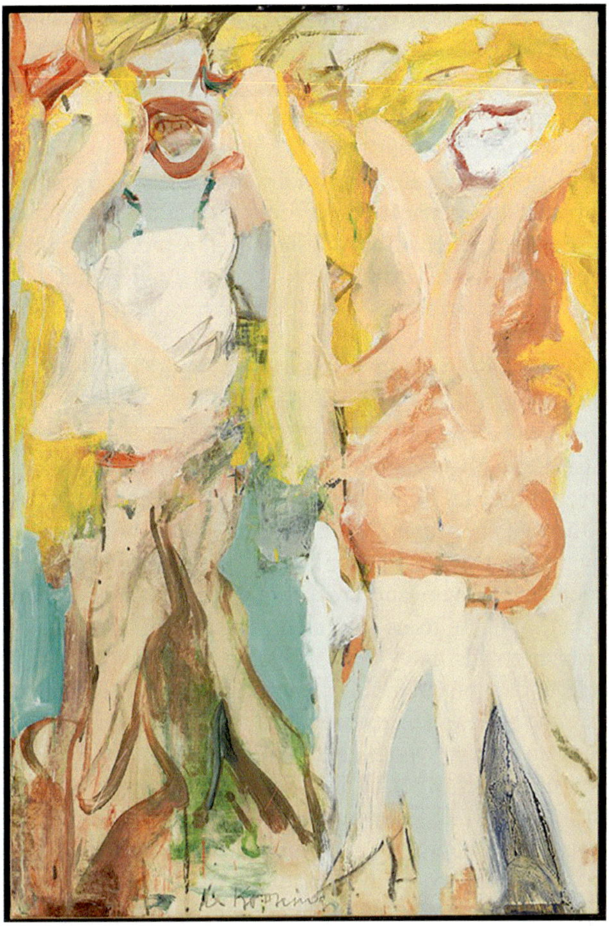

Figure 4.2 Willem de Kooning, *Women Singing II*, 1966. © Willem de Kooning Revocable Trust/ARS, NY and DACS, London 2025. Photo: Tate.

But the point I would make is this: The idea that vital to aesthetic response is the activation of embodied processes that replicate sensation as perceived in a work of art, the idea that activation of the motor system in the perception of art contributes significantly to aesthetic experience in which cognition is embodied as well, is truly limited. That the mirror neuron system (the interaction of brain cells stimulated in both the performance of a physical act and the viewing of someone else's performance of that act) is responsible for an embodiment constituting aesthetic experience is, in the context of the aesthetic, exceedingly narrow in scope. A "mediated intersubjectivity" – "a virtual, yet bodily-grounded as-if relation between the subjectivity of the beholder and that of the artist, encoded or evoked by the images' contents and/or by the artistic gestures that created the image"[10] – stresses simulation where *stimulation*, unequivocable and unequivocally, is what occurs. Gallese has seemingly qualified his thinking by claiming that the "relation between beholder and image is not interpersonal in a literal sense, but intersubjective by analogy," which removes the scientism from the theory. In hypothesizing that the intersubjectivity in question, the basis for embodied simulation, "activates the bodily and affective architecture through which intersubjectivity is enacted," he aims to qualify intersubjectivity, as he views it in aesthetic experience, as "[designating] a mode of embodied relation grounded in mechanisms that evolved for social interaction, but which can be re-directed toward cultural artifacts."[11] But does this really account for what occurs when one engages, for instance, with the David Smith painting or even that by De Kooning? Does this account for the association, the transformation, and inspiration that ensue from viewing these works?

Indeed, what is to be said of the mind's very capacity for imagining, the mind's ability to image? Does phantasia not throw into question the notion of embodied simulation which originates in the intentionality of perception, in the discernment of the object through the senses? What is to be said, moreover, of the space circumscribed by the creative imagination which entails entry into a field so resistant to representation as to circumvent any sort of cognitive knowing (however unconscious it may be)? What is to be said of the space circumscribed by the creative imagination which entails entry into a field so unrevealing of the gesture that engendered it as to circumvent motoric knowing? Is the sublime, with its resultant state of ekstasis, the only way to envision an adequate response to these questions?

Gallese states that "The hypothesis of embodied simulation proposes that the aesthetic power of images arises, at least in part, from their capacity to activate these pre-reflective, bodily-based mechanisms of understanding. Such mechanisms allow the viewer to internally re-enact, simulate, and thus 'feel into' the gesture, movement, or affect depicted in the image."[12] And if there is no image as such? Differentiated from shape and form, the image may be comprised of either or both, but is not reducible to either. What Gallese refers to as "oculocentrism" is indeed too restricted. And his challenging of the primacy of the visual brain in aesthetics is highly significant. But might suggestion – in the form of contraction and extension of the visible and the imperceptible, alterations in color and tone, and other impactful components as found, for example, in monochromatic paintings – not in some way impede bodily simulation to leave, yet again, the theoretician of aesthetic experience in too limited an arena? While she did not believe her painting monochromatic, the unifying sense emanating from a joining of tones, from an equilibration of color, provides many of the paintings of Geneviève Asse with a fullness that causes them to be seen as such. And, one wonders, might the visual processing of space, of the solid expanse of color often accompanied by the narrowest breakthrough of light, not defy, in its projection of quietude, the supposed source of empathic engagement and resultant neuronal activation of embodied simulation? Might the kind of neutrality found in her work not inhibit such a response in favor of one far less, if at all, "intersubjectively" and motorically determined?

Figure 4.3 Geneviève Asse © 2025 Artists Rights Society (ARS), New York / ADAGP, Paris

Given the neutrality of this painting, one even wonders where is the image. Is it really constricted to the edges of the canvas or does it extend beyond those limits? Certainly, there is nothing reproduced; yet nothing is negated. There is a sense of the comprehensive, the inclusive, yet nothing is made to appear. How is there a sense of containment with nothing contained? Is there, in fact, an image? If not, does that imply absence; does that signal emptiness? Does it even denote abstraction? Is the absence of figuration an expression, rather, of some sort of purity of the sensory? We look. And there is pleasure. Is the breakthrough of white – the PLAY of the spatial that keeps out the exterior while simultaneously letting it in, the PLAY of the temporal both spontaneous and structured – the source of that pleasure? Is the curiosity stimulated by the diminishing white, the SEEKING to know more, the source of that pleasure? Is it the color, with its subtle mixing of tones and their emotional resonance? Is there a resonance of one's "own motor representations of the same actions" with those of the painter, as Andy Clark describes embodied simulation?[13] There is, of course, the manifestation of the psychic unconscious both in the work of art and in its reception. In "Creative Writers and Day-Dreaming," Freud articulated the relation between fantasy or dream and literary creativity precisely in the context of unconscious wish-fulfillment. At the same time, however, it is important to recognize that he too claimed that "the wish makes use of an occasion in the present to construct, on the pattern of the past, a picture of the future,"[14] concomitantly pointing to prediction as well as to psychological motivation. But, once again, what of the "imageless image"?

One is reminded of the French philosopher Gilles Deleuze's articulation of the relation between painting and crisis: the need to go beyond the chaos of the "pre-pictorial" tumult of the modern world and generate what he called "a code for the future." Rejecting the chronology of figurative painting as preceding Expressionism and abstraction, he articulates an ethics of painting: "Why paint today?" To derive from the chaos and catastrophic disorder "a possible modern order."[15] Asse viewed painting in much the same way: Having been deeply involved in the Second World War as a volunteer ambulance driver, both with the Resistance and the French army, she viewed painting not as abstraction, but as a way of releasing the world from its contamination, of restoring to the world its fundamental simplicity, that of air and water and their ethically pure connotations.[16] Some situate the pleasure of her work therein.

Why the visual work of art (and the literary or musical work of art as well, though there are variations) offers what it does on the spectrum of pleasure is, in sum, a function of the interrelation of emotion with anticipation, of conscious awareness and cognition with sensorial perception, and even the modulation of neural activity by cultural influence. But there is also something more to be considered: The *what* in which this conjunction, this confluence, resides. And thus the question that imposes itself is this: Just what does the interrelation of thought and feeling, of perception and expectation, amount to, so to speak? Just what is the *being* of this work of art? Not only is there recognition of that which lays outside it and of the effect of that recognition on the uncertainty of the artwork. Not only is it poorly or beautifully executed. What is the nature of this artwork and what constitutes *experience* of it? Writing of the Dutch painter Geer van Velde, Beckett said this: "Believes painting should mind its own business, *i.e.* colour. *i.e.* no more say Picasso than Fabritius, Vermeer. Or inversely."[17] If we are to take Van Velde at his word – and Beckett's as well, for he too believed that painting (the purveyor of the "imageless image") did not transmit, any more than literary language, the external, the objectively real – what does "aesthetic experience" actually mean?

"Le Deuil de l'Objet" or The Ontology of Art

A non-deterministic perspective on the human psyche owed not only to constitutional and environmental factors (to genetics/epigenetics, disposition, and object relations), but also to drives (as Freud conceived of the term, though not limited to the two he described or even to the unconscious if one accepts Solms' idea of their being the "source of all consciousness"[18]), "becoming" puts the energic constitution of art, as of science, in high relief. It accounts for the experiential feature of predictive coding, for the tensions between expectation and surprise and their orientation toward the movement of time. It accounts for the developmental forward pull of maturation, which is to say that it accounts for individuation as phases rather than as an entity in and of itself. And it accounts for the resistance of matter to representation – what Beckett called, in a discussion of painting, "le deuil de l'objet" (the bereavement of the object)[19] – just as it accounts for the genesis of research as implicated in the quest for knowledge.

Observing a commonality between the phenomenology of Merleau-Ponty and the phenomenologically influenced (or, more precisely, Merleau-Pontian influenced) philosophy of Gilbert Simondon, Jacques Garelli writes of "the epistemology of microphysics [...] according to which we cannot radically separate the scientific 'object' discovered at the end of research from the path of the thought and operative processes that have led to revealing and constructing it."[20] Is the same not to be said of art? In comparing Simondon's critique of the "principle of individuation" with that of Merleau-Ponty, a critique laying forth the irreducibility of metastable systems to "the order of identity, unity, and alterity," Garelli describes the "tightly conjoined movement of being and of thought" which generates the "complex processes [...] that arise from a transindividual dimension of Being." He describes that which deconstructs the "corollaries" of that principle – "form, matter, substance, and fixed stable (autonomous) terms posited as realities-in-themselves" – and, "instead of reducing ontogenesis to the dimension restricted to and derived from the genesis of the individual," he confirms, citing Simondon, the need to confer onto the developmental process "the vaster characteristic of the 'becoming of being, that through which the being becomes insofar as it is, qua being.'"[21] If one could speak of individuation, one could as well speak of non-individuation or pre-individuation, Garelli, like Simondon, reasoned. Becoming and emergence, and thereby temporality, were the phenomenologically oriented contexts in which each considered the ontology of art, and the imaginative process, like the process of individuation, was for both a vital source of the renewal of one's sense of self.

Writing of the mid-20th-century painting identified as the École de Paris, and of the Abstract Expressionist painters in the United States at that time, Garelli described not only the ontological, but the proto-ontic (or pre-reflexive, antepredicative) order of the art in question and linked it with the works of several novelists as well. He emphasized what he termed the "preindividual horizon" from within which the painted forms, like characters and situations, progressively emerge. This dimension of the painting, like that of the novel, play, or poem, is the intertwining of the nascent individuations renewed with every viewing, every reading, as with every creative endeavor on the part of the artist, and it is this process of emergence, this movement of unfolding in space and time which evades any positivist, determinist identification that the reader or viewer may, however unaware, be pursuing.

A process of individuations, the artwork takes form, assumes meaning, by virtue of the shapes and images, the characterizations, which extend beyond the fixity, beyond the unity of identity and the habitual, to reveal its ontological charge and universality. In writing of the Italian philosopher Giambattista Vico, Beckett put it this way: "Individuality is the concretion of universality, and every individual action is at the same time superindividual. The individual and the universal cannot be considered as distinct from each other."[22] Critic Doris Hering said much the same when writing of the German expressionist dancer Dore Hoyer: Hoyer was "the essence of modern dance," or "movement rising from a deeply personal source to assume universality,"[23] with universality intended not as a minimization of individuality, but an enlargement within the transindividual process of perpetual becoming, the ontogenesis, of being.

Henri Maldiney was another, who, in the tradition of French phenomenology, spoke of art and, in particular, of painting as a "field of tensions," a rhythm. "Maldiney takes us out of a philosophy of consciousness," notes Eliane Escoubas, "[…] to substitute for it a philosophy of presence. ('Being there.')." Pointing to the difference between "presence" and representation, as Maldiney defined it, Escoubas observes that the word "presence" – *praesens* in Latin – means being before oneself. "Exist" means the same, with the Latin *existere/exsistere* meaning "to come into view, appear, show oneself, come into being." Thus, she concludes, "This is why art that presents, and does not represent, is 'existential,' like man. Man and the work of art ex-ist."[24] Ascribing this existential phenomenon that is art, this individuating process that is the aesthetic, to corporeal subjectivity, Merleau-Ponty went so far as to claim that one does not inhabit one's body but experiences by way of the body and, he claimed, "It is by lending his body to the world that the artist changes the world into paintings."[25] In this statement, he is no further removed than Maldiney from Freud's recognition of the bodily surface as "a place from which both external and internal perceptions may spring," no further removed from Freud's idea that it is through the body, psychophysiologically speaking, through the mental projection of its surface, that the ego itself arises.

Contrary to any purely conceptualizing perspective, to any logical or semiotic understanding of aesthetic experience – in light of the preindividual, of individuations in formation, of a transcendental landscape generating form and meaning – art, in a word, is replete with tension, contrast, and nuance and cannot be reduced to anything external to it in as much as it abounds with potential, with possibility. And it is *emergence*, that which not only defies the fixating logic of identifying symbolization, the determinism of the re-presentational, that allows for feeling and, consequentially, meaning to be created.[26] In demonstrating how obsolete is the hylomorphic principle of individuation, in demonstrating the need for awareness of the processes intrinsic to the formations of individuals, formations "never completed, never fixed, never stable, but always accomplishing in their evolution an individuation that structures them, without these individuals fully eliminating the associated charge of pre-individuality," Garelli, like

Merleau-Ponty before him, articulates the "individualizing movement of knowledge" that is simultaneously a "movement of being."[27] In so doing, he elucidates the meaning of transduction, defined as "a form-taking in conjunction with the energetic discharge of the metastable system that is revealed as being more than unity and more than identity."[28] In so doing, he underscores Simondon's emphasis on "the incompetence of the principle of identity."[29] And, in so doing, he reveals the meeting of art and science in the acknowledgment of "the dominant state of nature [as] not matter but energy,"[30] in the philosophy of being.

Framing "the usage of theories borrowed from thermodynamics and quantum physics in the philosophical problematic of the pre-individual and the contemporary conception of beings" led Garelli to the "pressing question" posed by Werner Heisenberg to Niels Bohr cited previously. We recall that these two physicists, for whom "the philosophical status (but which could also be called the 'mode of being') of the quantum particle" was primary, bemoaned the lack of a means (a "language") to "deal with" the understanding of atoms, and that Bohr, as reported by Heisenberg, said the real meaning of "understanding" was needed as a result. If Bohr and Heisenberg considered the "mode of being" of the quantum particle, so must the aesthetician consider the "mode of being" of the work of art. What does "understanding" in the aesthetic context mean? Placing the image (visual or other) outside the domain of cognition, far from what Lisa Feldman Barrett and others consider preliminary to its creation, situating its ontology between subject and object in a zone of immediacy and intuition, is how Henri Bergson, another for whom the "way of thinking" and "what is to be thought" were inseparable, considered art. An "anti-concept," as Bruno Clément calls it when writing of Bergson, art is linked with science, with the biological sciences more specifically, the one shedding light upon the other in a mutuality of anti-materialistic, anti-deterministic finalism: "le caractère d'imprévisibilité du devenir" (the unpredictability of becoming) being the touchstone of the one as of the other. Art, associable with science by virtue of its examination of life, goes beyond intelligence for Bergson, however, and is not understandable as a divisible and decomposable object, simply because the intuition which gave rise to it is unanalyzable for being in perpetual evolution.[31]

Most recently, Shaun Gallagher has similarly explained "understanding" with an emphasis on the cognitive recognized not merely as an event of the brain, but as embodied, as emerging "from processes distributed across brain-body-environment," which is to say, an emphasis on the world as apprehended, not as "pre-given." For Gallagher, cognitive processes are to be understood "in view of their role in worldly contexts where they acquire meaning rather than as a representational mapping or replicated internal model of the world." It is the very notion of representation, according to Gallagher, that deflects from our comprehension of cognition as shaped by bodily affect (whether hunger and fatigue or mood and emotion) and contingent upon social and intersubjective conditions.[32]

Already in Freud we find evidence of the embodiment of mind and its negation of our "understanding" the world as a phenomenon independent of such conditions. Offering a drawing of the "structural relations" of the mind (those of the id, ego, and super-ego), Freud noted the insufficiency of linear outlines to depict the intangible processes of psychic function, of personality and its dynamic constitution. For the more accurate depiction of the merging of super-ego into the id, of the movement of separation and integration, of regressions and returns of the ever mobile ego, the very mobility of the constituents of the mind must be made to appear. And to this end he specified the need for "areas of colour melting into one another as they are presented by modern artists."[33] Perhaps the work of no modern artist illustrates this "melting" of color and the intangibility and movement of the mind that it projects as much as that of Mark Rothko. The immediacy of the areas of color in Rothko's work, their radiance and affective impact, reveal the energy constituting mental function. This is particularly so of the paintings of the late 1950s and 1960s when form (which is not to say image) became this artist's principal preoccupation and primary means of color projection. If not the structure of the mind, if not the relations sketched by Freud in the effort to reveal the components of personality, what Rothko's work lays bare is the mind's vitality. In so doing, paintings such as "Orange and Yellow" reveal the immateriality of art, its intangibility, and, thereby, the very nature of its being.

In looking at Rothko's earlier paintings, however, one has a different kind of experience. In fact, one might be inclined to see in some a resemblance to the lone self-portrait painted by the artist in 1936. One might even be repeatedly startled by the appearance, in each of the figurations, inexact as they are, of facial congruities, likenesses to the geometry of Rothko's own face. The triangular, circular, rectangular forms: all might be viewed as projecting, in multiple viewings spread over time, a similitude that leads one to think more about the notions put forth by some of the cognitively oriented neuroscientists and aestheticians mentioned in the previous chapter. I brought this (my own experience) to Rothko's son, Christopher Rothko, who reacted thus: "I think if you are seeing these hidden figures, you are perhaps looking at the works too closely. My father's works are gestalts, works to be *experienced* rather than seen. He is having a conversation with the viewer, based on a shared experience of the human condition. That is the starting point, and of course, the interaction will become far more specific and personal with each viewer and each encounter."[34]

Such a juxtaposition of "experience" and "seeing" implies a dichotomy of the very sort that Merleau-Ponty, Garelli, Simondon, Maldiney, and Bergson all aimed, in one way or another, to unravel. Are the energic nature of experience and the fluidity of perception, such as in the act of seeing, not deeply intertwined? Irreducible to the rational, to the core element of the Cartesian, "seeing" is inseparable from the "experience" of recognition or the lack thereof, inseparable from emotion and its influence on the brain's combinatory responsiveness to the vision at hand. Does "seeing" necessarily imply the reading into a work of "understanding" when this or that impression or interpretation was unintended by the artist? Is "seeing" a function of cognition imposed as familiarity upon an otherwise unfamiliar terrain? Perhaps most significant, is the ontological dimension of the aesthetic experience somehow disrupted by an artist's visual identification of themselves, no matter how minimal and one of which they were consciously unaware? Might what I refer to as the "imageless image" be a capturing of that very dimension?

In the context of painters who have sought – whether through a more suggestive if distorted allusion to the external or a very deliberate depiction of the total absence of the object world – to create the "imageless image," Agnes Martin, once again, immediately comes to mind. As noted previously, one enters the arena of a Martin painting to relate to what she referred to as her "inspiration." And one does so by way of the absence, not the presence, of the identifiable (which is to say the presence, as in Beckett, of the absence). In the paintings created after 1974, after a seven-year hiatus from artmaking, one sees an increase in the level of abstraction and the value that "inspiration" had for Martin. Having destroyed her early work, which was more figurative, and having gone through an exploratory period in which she delved deeply into the relation between vertical and horizontal planes, Martin became increasingly mobile in her work, increasingly free of the constraints imposed by the dichotomy of subject and object. Cerebration no longer appeared in her painting as it had in the exploration with horizontal and vertical lines, with planes of color and divisions of space, but a way of being in the world, a way of being *of* the world, as Merleau-Ponty would have it, is what became dominant. This ontological uniformity of ego and world would implicate a manner of looking at the work, a manner of "seeing" both for the painter and those viewing it. This was the "starting point" for Martin.

Claiming, as she often did, that art has its source in "inspiration," Martin referred to the revelations that came to her when she closed herself off to the world, when solitude provided the means for her to open herself to the reverie-like activity not unlike that of free association such as it occurs in the consulting room. This is the place, the internal space, in which form, she would say, yields to formlessness, the stasis of imaging to the activity of imagining. "My paintings have neither object nor space nor line nor anything – no forms," she wrote. "They are light, lightness, about merging, about formlessness, breaking down form."[35] The notion of formlessness, linked to what I call the "imageless image," is stunningly reminiscent of Merleau-Ponty's citation of poet Paul Valéry in "The Eye and the Mind": "The painter 'takes his body with him,' says Valéry." "Indeed," Merleau-Ponty continues, "we cannot imagine how a *mind* could paint." And, once again, "It is by lending his body to the world that the artist changes the world into paintings."[36] Here again, as well, is Martin: "You wouldn't think of form by the ocean. You can go in if you don't encounter anything. A world without objects, without interruption, making a work without interruption or obstacle. It is to accept the necessity of the simple direct going into a field of vision as you would cross an empty beach to look at the ocean."[37]

"Minds are marvelous to look at from the inside."[38] It is hard to imagine a more apt expression of the neuropsychoanalytic subscription, based on Freud's own, to the necessity of viewing the phenomenon of mentation both subjectively as well as objectively. These words of Daniel Wegner would appear to underscore Martin's devotion to what she termed "inspiration," her devotion to a mind free of "[c]oncepts, relationships, categories, classifications, [and] deductions." "There are two parts of the mind," she wrote. "The outer mind that records facts and the inner mind that says 'yes' and 'no.' When you think of something that you should do, the inner mind says 'yes' and you feel elated. We call this inspiration. For an artist this is the only way."[39]

But inspiration for Martin was not only about submission, about *having* to turn the "little picture" she had in her mind "into a six-foot canvas."[40] It was also about the universality of certain kinds of experience, experience that was unencumbered by personal feelings or cognitive intrusions. Happiness, for instance, or other "states that transcend the particular conditions of an individual life," as art critic Nancy Princenthal has put it, were what qualified as art for Martin. And thus her paintings, especially those of her later years, aimed to elicit from the viewer the response one has before nature: "There's nobody living who couldn't stand all afternoon in front of a waterfall. It's a simple experience, you become lighter and lighter in weight… Anyone who can sit on a stone in a field a while can see my painting. Nature is like parting a curtain, you go into it." Martin wanted "to draw a certain response like this" from the viewer, "that quality of response from people when they leave themselves behind."[41] This is what Rothko, and the Abstract Expressionist more generally, continually sought in wanting their "works to be *experienced* rather than seen."

Art, for Martin, was first and foremost about beauty, the beauty that resides not within the work itself but within the mind that apprehends it: "When a beautiful rose dies, beauty does not die because it is not really in the rose. Beauty is an awareness in the mind. It is a mental and emotional response that we make."[42] Or, as her gallerist and longtime friend Arne Glimcher tells it, "My granddaughter Isabelle visited Agnes in New Mexico in the early 1990s. During that visit, Agnes took a rose from a vase and holding it out towards Isabelle asked if the Rose was beautiful. 'Yes,' Isabelle replied. Agnes then put the rose behind her back and asked if the rose was still beautiful. Again Isabelle said yes to the rose now hidden behind Agnes. She demonstrated to a child that the concept of beauty was only in the mind not in the object."[43]

Martin's notion of art as existing in the mind of the viewer as opposed to the artwork – "Everybody's got their mind on artists and paintings," she claimed. "But it's the *response* to art that really matters"[44] – is best appreciated, I would argue, in the context of the "imageless image," whether in Martin's work or in the kind of abstraction, of absence even, found as well in the art of others (writers, choreographers, and composers alike). I would cite once again in this regard Shaun Gallagher who has written of the sublime as an overwhelming of the imagination in a way that describes one's connection with the paintings of Martin, Rothko, and others: "Perhaps the most important thing to be said about the sublime," claims Gallagher, "is what we cannot say. The notion of the sublime includes the idea that it is something that *cannot be represented*."[45] So, too, we recall in this regard the "oceanic" feeling that the writer Romain Rolland famously wrote about to Freud and that Freud described in terms of "limitlessness," of "a bond with the universe," and the "oneness" of the infant with the world, an intimacy designated the "primary ego-feeling" in 1930 in *Civilization and Its Discontents*.[46]

Even in paintings where the transcendence of the sublime, the wholeness of the oceanic, and the feelings associated with one or the other prevail – paintings so highly abstract as to reveal only color and form, only the uniqueness of the "imageless image" – a bodily manifestation is present. It is present in what Samuel Abrams called the "forward pull" of human development. It is present in what Doris Hering referred when writing of the "essence of modern dance." It is present in the process of transindividuation, the pre-reflexive and antepredicative process delineated by Garelli and Simondon in their writings on the energic transformations constituting the creation and reception of art. It is present in the "arising of external and internal perceptions" from one's body demarcated by Freud as the source of the ego. And it is present in the non-descriptive "understanding" of the atom as well.

As though responding to Heisenberg's and Bohr's concern with the "'mode of being' of the quantum particle" and with the lack of a "language" to describe it, Garelli wrote of the creative unfolding of the artwork as congruent with a process, a spatiotemporal "mondification" ("worldification") process irreducible to the order of communication. In his discussion of the movement, the emergence, integral to the visual as to the literary work of art, he captures what Martin, like other of her contemporaries, sought to reveal: not the visible, but the coming to be seen. "There is a paradox of poetic activity," to cite once again Garelli's explanation regarding the example of poetry, "that is the measure of its condition. Opening onto the world, the poem is, in the act of unveiling, that which is unveiled. A gaze, it makes itself seen. Light, it illuminates itself. Revealer, it reveals only in being itself revealed."[47] Samuel Beckett's entire oeuvre is a case in point.

In the continual focus on the creation of the image in his plays, novels, and poems, Beckett seeks to unveil in what aesthetic experience consists. His writing consistently centers on the boundaries of language, on rhetorical failure, and the irresolvable problem posed by representation. "L'objet de la représentation résiste toujours à la représentation" ("the object of representation always resists representation"), he wrote of painting.[48] And this of literature:

> Is there any reason why that terrible materiality of the word surface should not be capable of being dissolved, like for example the sound surface, torn by enormous pauses, of Beethoven's seventh Symphony, so that through whole pages we can perceive nothing but a path of sounds suspended in giddy heights, linking unfathomable abysses of silence?[49]

In his effort to transmit the impossibility of transmitting the visual verbally, of uncovering what lies behind the "materiality of the word surface" and achieving a "literature of the unword,"[50] Beckett sought to reveal that which is the impediment of sight. He sought to reveal figuration of the object as comparable to words themselves, painting as comparable to literature in its failure to re-present the unrepresentable. If the functional and dynamic was Freud's way of moving from the topological and anatomical to the mental, the subversion of language – the attempt to expose the materiality of the word and the futility of its undoing – was Beckett's way of exposing both its *potential* and failure to mean.[51]

In both his critical writings and his literary texts, Beckett recognized the limits of expression and favored the challenge to closure that abstract art, visual or literary, revealed. Imagining for Beckett meant pursuing the quest for the unwording of literature, for words (like the unrepresentable object) dim the view: "Less. Less seen. Less seeing. Less seen and seeing when with words than when not," we read in *Worstward Ho*.[52] Language as representation is tried and shown consistently to fail. Beckett's unwording of literature resembles highly abstract visual art where there is no image, as such, to see. Just as the painting of Rothko, of Martin, and others *reveals seeing itself*, with all the contextualizing that affect, localization, and more bring to bear on the viewing of the imageless work, just as the object conceals and refuses re-presentation in their painting, words for Beckett are impediments. (It was not for nothing that Beckett's 1948 essay on the brothers Geer and Bram van Velde, Dutch painters whose work Beckett highly valued for its refusal to yield to the subject-object dichotomy, is titled "Peintres de l'empêchement.") It is a comparable dynamic, a similar *virtuality* or *capacity* for meaning, as opposed to its actualization, that is evident in the late prose works, such as *Ill Seen Ill Said* and *Worstward Ho*, where recapitulation prevents the tracing of a linear or anecdotal (in other words, narrative and thereby representational) progression. For seeing, like Freud's dynamic, like Freud's functional emphasis on association, is of the mind. "Imagination Dead Imagine" Beckett – ironically, but not *so* ironically – titled a prose text in 1965 and *Stirrings Still* (1989) his final prose work. Included in his 1979 text *Company*, appears the following:

> This at first sight seems clear. But as the eye dwells it grows obscure. Indeed the longer the eye dwells the obscurer it grows. Till the eye closes and freed from pore the mind inquires, What does this mean? What does this mean that at first sight seemed clear? [...] Pangs of faint light and stirrings still. Unformulable gropings of the mind. Unstillable.[53]

Forever in search of the stabilizing solution to the potentially critical disruption brought about by surprise and uncertainty, Beckett imagined when words failed. Poems, plays, novels: "Ever tried. Ever failed. No matter. Try again. Fail again. Fail better."[54] Famous words from *Worstward Ho*. One thinks of his early work for the theater: *Endgame* where two of the actors are in garbage cans. Or his somewhat later one-act theater piece entitled *Play* where three characters interact from within funeral urns. Indelible visual images (made all the more indelible by his detailed scenic instructions and his steadfast insistence on their being adhered to) enduring over and above any verbal iteration, but images of those on the verge of not being, which is precisely where Beckett himself was when he composed his last piece of writing.

"What is the Word" is a poem that most explicitly, if paradoxically, displays the very coming into being of the image which, by virtue of the failure of language, is but glimpsed:

> [...]
> seeing –
> folly seeing all this –
> this –
> what is the word –
> this this –
> this this here –
> all this this here –
> folly given all this –
> seeing –
> folly seeing all this this here –
> for to –
> what is the word –
> see –
> glimpse –
> seem to glimpse –
> need to seem to glimpse –
> folly for to need to seem to glimpse –
> what –
> what is the word –
> [...][55]

At this time it was not only "the materiality of the word surface" that interfered with the emergence of the image from language. Beckett's failure to find the word, however "material" its surface, is said to have been the result of damage to his brain. In 1988, following a fall that left him unconscious, Beckett underwent hospital tests that did not definitively determine whether he had suffered a stroke, had Parkinson's disease, or it was some other neurological cause that was responsible for what Laura Salisbury has described as the writer's experiencing of "a temporary yet debilitating aphasia."[56] As described by Salisbury, "What is the Word" is "[s]cattered with stuttered dashes, abrupt elisions, compulsive repetitions and controlled echoes that inhabit an uncanny hinterland between the voluntary and the involuntary" and, most interestingly, she offers this:

> Although the biography is clear that there is a firm connection between the inception of "What Is the Word" and aphasia, it seems significant that neither critics at the time, nor those since, have read or registered this final work as the expression of a disabled author. One simple explanation for this is that 'What Is the Word' is not Beckett in any recognisably "defective" mode, distanced from his previous style and central concerns. [...] Here, what is left of a perceiving being is thrown amidst a thickened and resistant material world that will not yield to either naming or comprehension, as language becomes a crust of material signifiers that occludes representation.

And, in line with the above, this:

> The fact that there is something that feels lost in this world of banal material signifiers that refuse to be bound to their signifieds endows the poem with an affective quality; indeed, it materialises affect as a witness to linguistic privation.[57]

It was apropos of the resistance of the material to representation that Beckett wrote (once again, ironically, but not *so* ironically) of "le deuil de l'objet" (the bereavement of the object) in painting. And pitting the ontic against the ontological is how one might describe his own play (or PLAY) with presence and absence, with the representation of the un-representable.

Beckett's writings on painting ("La peinture des van Velde ou le monde et le pantalon," written soon after the Second World War, and "Peintres de l'empêchement" which dates to 1948, among others) presaged Merleau-Ponty's 1961 essay "Eye and Mind" which begins with the following sentence: "Science manipulates things and gives up living in them." The philosopher's text continues as a plea for a return from the absolutism of the laboratory, from a thinking so "operationally" deterministic as to have "become a sort of absolute artificialism, such as we see in the ideology of cybernetics, where human creations are derived from a natural information process, itself conceived on the model of human machines." And then with a warning: "If this kind of thinking were to extend its dominion over humanity and history; and if, ignoring what we know of them through contact and our own situations, it were to set out to construct them on the basis of a few abstract indices [...] then, since the human being truly becomes the *manipulandum* he thinks he is, we enter into a cultural regimen in which there is neither truth nor falsehood concerning humanity and history, into a sleep, or nightmare from which there is no awakening." Merleau-Ponty was advocating for a kind of scientific thinking wherein there would be a "return to the 'there is' which precedes it; to the site, the soil of the sensible and humanly modified world such as it is in our lives and for our bodies – not that possible body which we may legitimately think of as an information machine but this actual body I call mine, this sentinel standing quietly at the command of my words and my acts."[58]

Like Beckett, Merleau-Ponty was dedicated to revealing the relation between word and object, a relation he described as chiasmic. And he stressed embodiment as the way into perception. If disembodiment – whether the disembodied cry of *Breath* or the disembodied self of *Not I*, to name but two – takes center stage throughout Beckett's oeuvre, it is that nothing is not nothing in Beckett's literary art any more than in the philosophical writing of his phenomenological contemporary. Rather than focusing on intentionality, the subject's projection toward the object of perception (Husserl), or on the notion of being-in-the-world (Heidegger), Merleau-Ponty and Beckett were primarily concerned with the bodily experience through which sensorial apperception and its conscious or unconscious registering occur. And art was congruent for both with the ontology of that non-objectifiable experience, with its at once non-conceptualizable and revelatory nature. If Beckett disavowed any connection with philosophy (whether existential, the perspective with which he was often aligned, or any other), it was not that he did not recognize a relation between the visual or literary and the philosophical. Rather, it was that that relation was irreducible to intellectualization. It was that that relation was manifested in the experiential encounter from which art is created, in the *waiting* for Godot, the *searching* for "the Word," the *listening* to Krapp's last tape in the play of that name. All was to be written, for the writer's creativity resides in what critic Enoch Brater has called "the terrifying necessity of writing *things* down, whatever the word is or whatever that record becomes." As Brater says, "How the 'word' is now heard – and precisely *what* that word *is* – depends for its life on the personality who delivers 'all this this here – .' *This* can only be the sound of a word in the listener's private vocabulary of tone and mood and gesture." The performer, the listener, the viewer, the word: "[W]hat a fertile laboratory," Brater concludes, is the drama in Beckett's text.[59]

"Fertile," indeed, as owed to the very process of association whereby the attribution of meaning, as owed to the ontology of art whence the drama. It is the ontological grounding of the aesthetic, rather than its ontic reification in the literary text, the painting, theatrical script, or musical score, *the mode of existence of art as opposed to representation in the artwork*, that is dramatic in itself. In an appendix to his 1915 paper "The Unconscious," an appendix entitled "Words and Things," Freud wrote that "there corresponds to the word a complicated associative process." He explains this by distinguishing the "word-presentation," which is "seen to be something closed, even though capable of extension," from the "object-presentation," which he describes as "not closed" and linked to the "word-presentation" through its acquisition of meaning. And he describes the former as made up of "sound-image," "visual letter-image," "motor speech-image," and "motor writing-image" while the latter is "a complex of associations made up of the greatest variety of visual, acoustic, tactile, kinaesthetic and other presentations."[60] Whether termed "object presentation" or "thing presentation" as Freud also referred to it, the point is that the work of art is irreducible to its thingness; it is irreducible either to the object that "presents" it or to the image(s) that it presents. As Beckett observed, "Being is constantly putting form in danger."[61] And it is this that is projected in the most abstract of paintings.

If certain of the conclusions regarding the application of predictive coding to painting are problematic, as I have argued, they are all the more so when one considers that we do not look at a painting in the same way we look at objects. A painting is not viewed in space any more than the literary text we read or the symphony we hear.

> This leads to two alternative interim conclusions. The more radical and (skeptical) one suggests that the PEM account of real-world perception [...] is incompatible with a deep experience of a work of art [...]. Accordingly, the basic tenet of the Bayesian framework that the brain minimizes unpredictability is at odds with the ontological nature of works of art, which defy predictability. The less radical and more accommodating option suggests that the deeper experience of works of art requires that viewers be able to tune or adapt their prediction mechanisms to the specific visual environment of the museum [...].[62]

Freud's well-known 1920 description of his grandson's utterances of *fort* ("Gone!") and *da* ("There!") while playing, while tossing a small object into hiding and subsequently pulling it back into sight, gave rise to a variety of interpretations of the infantile psyche and some, like Melanie Klein and Donald Winnicott, were inspired by it to develop play techniques for therapy with children. Whether of the child's pain at separation from his mother or of the world into which he was thrown without her, mastery has explained the pleasure of the game. The original discussion by Freud actually focused on two games, each related to a different moment, but both having to do with disappearance and reappearance, both relating not only to the possibility of return, of continuity, of attainment, in other words, of the symbolic order, but to the *sentience of the imaginative order*, the pleasure inherent in *imagining* the turn of absence into presence.

This interplay of absence and presence has provided many an artist with a contextual frame for the creative endeavor. In fact, applicable to all works of art, it is precisely this that supplies the *rhythm* essential to aesthetic form, by which I mean the arrangement in time and space of the creative act and that of the engagement of reader, viewer, or listener as well. To put it otherwise, there is a rhythm definable not only as the sonorous dimension, for instance, of a musical work itself, but as the spatiotemporal dimension of the acts of composing and listening, as of writing and reading and painting and viewing. And it is this rhythm, the rhythm of creativity and receptivity, that is overlooked by those attending to recognition and the lack thereof in the work of art whatever the genre. The idea that aesthetic pleasure results from the minimization of prediction error, from the succession of more unpredictability to less uncertainty and the pleasure that lies therein, like the reductionistic perspective of psychobiography (as we shall see in Chapter Five) and other deterministic perspectives, disregards that very rhythm to the detriment of the ontology of aesthetic experience. If the notions of the ontological and related individualizing horizons of the artwork – horizons from within which emerges aesthetic form – preempt a conceptual means of grasping the meaning of aesthetic experience, so, too, the participatory states of both creator and receptor, irreducible to the cognitive apprehension of art offered by recognition, are part of the empirical rhythm that cannot be ignored. And it shares with psychoanalysis – with the transference upon which its very process depends, with the regression that will culminate in an "emotional reintegration," as Gilbert Rose refers to it – an ontological dimension owed to the creative imagination.

"Ontological Psychoanalysis"

The "primitive edge of experience" is a term introduced by Thomas Ogden in his account of the early organization of the psyche. Along with the depressive and paranoid-schizoid positions (as conceived by Melanie Klein) and what Ogden calls the "autistic-contiguous mode," experience is generated, Ogden maintains, by way of the interplay between these earliest phases of development. Unlike those of Freud or Klein, whose views of psychological organization (whether in terms of sexual pleasure or the need for human contact) explain behavior, Ogden's focus is not only on consequential behavior, but the interdependence of experiential qualities. And, specifically, it is the autistic-contiguous position or phase of infancy that – "as a sensory-dominated, presymbolic area of experience in which the most primitive form of meaning is generated on the basis of the organization of sensory impressions" – is of relevance here.[63]

The relevance of the autistic-contiguous position, defined by Ogden as the time of the infant's most primitive efforts to create "a sense of boundedness for his sensory experience,"[64] resides, on the one hand, in its domination by the sensory and, on the other, in the sense of coherence for which it strives. This is to say that this earliest phase of infancy, which has features such as "shape, hardness, coldness, warmth, and texture"[65] that constitute feeling and thereby the earliest sense of self, is neither solely biologically nor environmentally determined. It is a feeling phase which illustrates the emanation of consciousness, "becoming mind," for the infant would not "know" it was experiencing such features and express desire (wanting to nurse, for example) or distress (when needing to be held). It is a grounding phase, a phase in which the integration of drives, their reconciliation, begins to take hold. And it is a phase which serves to "[ward] off anxiety related to the disruption of the sensory-dominated, rudimentary sense of self," as Ogden makes known by case presentations illustrating "the anxiety of disintegration" one may later encounter – the fear, if not of an actual *crisis* of mental health, a *crisis* "on the primitive edge of experience" – when one aims precisely to reestablish the "continuity of the bounded sensory surface."[66] It is this notion of destabilization and reintegration that brings to our attention a kind of congruence between aesthetic experience and psychoanalytic process. But to grasp the import of that congruence and what it revels of the meaning of form we need to look at Ogden's idea of what he calls "ontological psychoanalysis."

Ogden uses the term "ontological psychoanalysis" "to refer," as he has written, "to a dimension of psychoanalysis in which the analyst's primary focus is on facilitating the patient's efforts to become more fully himself."[67] Shifting from an emphasis on knowing, on insight and understanding, an epistemological emphasis primarily attributable to Freud and Klein, to an emphasis *on being and becoming*, an ontological perspective to which Wilfred Bion and Donald Winnicott are considered to have been the primary contributors, Ogden is far from minimizing the value for Freud and Klein of ontology and that for Bion and Winnicott of the epistemophilic. He does, however, seek to demonstrate, over and above their interconnection, less the value of understanding than the creative experience of its achievement, less the epistemological dimension involving the arrival at "understandings of previously unconscious thoughts, feelings, and bodily experience, which help the patient achieve psychic change" than the ontological dimension that involves "providing an interpersonal context in which forms of experiencing, states of being, come to life in the analytic relationship that were previously unimaginable by the patient (for instance, the states of being involved in *experiencing* transitional objects and phenomena" and "in experiencing the silent communication at the core of the self'"[68]). "*Wo Es war, soll Ich werden*: Where id [it] was, there ego [I] shall be"[69] is cited by Ogden in light of Freud's own ontological thinking in the sense that "[w]hat had been experienced as other to oneself ('the it') is incorporated into one's being (who I am, who I 'shall *be*,' who I am becoming."[70]

As Jules Kerman has said of Ogden's ontological analysis, "all is in the moment and is becoming." It is something similar, I would venture, that nears the ontology of psychoanalysis to the ontology of art: In designating this new sensibility "ontological," a reference to what is "being" or emerging ("becoming"), Ogden aims, writes Kerman, "to pull us away" from the notion of mind "as 'apparatus,'" to have us think of it, rather, "as process, continuous 'dreaming,' toward what poetry or great fiction, music, or art offer access."[71] Similarly, Rose describes the aesthetic experience as "the opportunity for regression and/or progression, 'escape' or expansion in a dynamically changing 'living' balance." Where the aesthetic experience and the psychoanalytic process resonate, according to Rose, is in the affording of intense or "dangerous degrees of affect" and "integration [...] within the safe holding presence" that each not only arouses, but encourages.[72] The shared result entails an objectivation of form, "sentient patterns of tension and release that elicit a responsive *resonance* of corresponding tension and release experienced subjectively as emotion." And even more to the point, "the establishment and organization of perceptual tensions in the artwork are so finely tuned that it offers an objective image of apparent attunement to the experience of human feelings."[73]

In this correspondence between aesthetic experience and psychoanalytic process, a subliminal correspondence emanating from the ontology of each accounts for the essence of creativity. Perception and sentience are the biological ingredients of form and, once again, as in the consideration of SEEKING and PLAY, we come to the emanation of creativity from the drive to know. We come to imagination, to the creation of order and form, from engagement with the unknown. We come to imagination by way of curiosity and experimentation (the pleasurable "what if" of PLAY), which is to say that we come to the site where art meets science. It is at this very site that Freud joins Panksepp and Solms and, ultimately, with the formation of prediction the result of memory and expectation, Friston as well.

As previously noted, Freud offers in *The Ego and the Id* a unique illustration of the ontological dimension that removes art from the material, from its designation as matter, as "object," and thereby a way into the understanding of aesthetic experience. His distinction between the descriptive and dynamic – between the illustrative and the functional – comes to the fore with the body serving as the principal focus of the distinction. In *From Neurology to Psychoanalysis: Sigmund Freud's Neurological Drawings and Diagrams of the Mind*, Lynn Gamwell and Mark Solms declare that "the fact that the ego derives from 'a mental projection of the surface of the body' cannot be overestimated" and that this reiteration of what had been described earlier by Freud, the idea "that higher cortical networks transform information derived from the body periphery until it is so altered that it can no longer be reasonably described in anatomical terms," attests to a transformation that "*is the origin of the mind.*" Citing Freud's work *On Aphasia* published in 1891, they note that "The ego, too, therefore, could ultimately be said to 'contain the body periphery in the same way as a poem contains the alphabet, in a complete rearrangement, serving different purposes.'"[74] Their point is that what occurs is not a straightforward projection onto the cortex of the body periphery but, rather, an implementing of a functional as opposed to a topological connection between the two. It is with this understanding, they claim, that "the *mind* – that aspect of the organism which represents the body not concretely but rather *functionally, abstractly and symbolically* – entered Freud's scientific work."[75] Of particular interest here is the idea that *no more than the body, which is not directly imprinted on the cortex, is psychology concretely projected onto anatomy or the poem, akin to both, plotted onto letters of the alphabet.*

In citing the poem's relation to the alphabet as analogous to the ego's relation to the body, Freud was underscoring, if not defining, the very nature of the experiential. Already, when explaining in an 1888 medical dictionary article entitled "Aphasie" that "A 'word' is not a simple idea, but a complex that consists of four elements, two sensory and two motor," he did not delineate in any detail the components before stressing that "the connections that link the four elements of the word presentation with *the idea of the object* must be taken into consideration."[76] On the brink of delineating the psychological, he was on the verge, however unintentionally, of articulating *the very nature of experience*: ideational or imagistic as well as any other. Not endorsing either of his teacher Theodor Meynert's models of psychic functioning, neither the anatomical nor physiological, he viewed the mental "independently of their organic substrates," as the translators/editors of the neuroscientific article on aphasia concluded.[77] Warning the reader of *On Aphasia* against "[mistaking] the scaffolding for the building," Freud would be careful, they wrote, to avoid "the temptation to determine psychical locality in any anatomical fashion." Instead, they explained, he would "remain upon psychological ground" and proposed that we "picture the instrument which carries out our mental functions as resembling a compound microscope or a photographic apparatus, or something of the kind. On that basis, psychical locality [would] correspond to a point inside the apparatus at which one of the preliminary stages of *an image comes into being*."[78]

Functional or dynamic, as contrasted with topological or anatomical, was Freud's way from the physiological to the psychological, the way into the mental. Concomitantly, I would argue, it provides a way into the creative: While there would be no creativity without the contribution of the neocortex, as Panksepp has said, "there are no intrinsic urges for creativity in the cortex itself."[79] And just as there would be "no fine arts, music, dance, or engaging stories without the enthusiastic appetitive arousals of the healthy human SEEKING system" – in other words, without curiosity – "[t]here would be few stories and songs if our creative juices were not stirred by powerful affective tides within the emotional fabrics of our minds." Thus Panksepp's conclusion that "Emotional feelings are foundational for all the arts,"[80] which pertains, of course, to the viewer, listener, or reader as well as the creator themselves.

I have thus far sought to situate aesthetic experience in terms of drive, in terms that go beyond the libidinal and aggressive categories foundational in Freud to include curiosity and creativity as emanating from the emotional drive systems of SEEKING and PLAY and the predictive processing that enframes them. I noted in this regard (in Chapter Two) the curiosity-evoking title of some of Geneviève Asse's paintings, "Fenêtre" ("Window"), and its applicability to all her work in accordance with Silvia Baron Supervielle's commentary. And I have stressed the relation of this feature, this enticement, to the arousal of the SEEKING system, to the active engagement with uncertainty, with the unknown that defines it. This enticement, however, is but one manifestation of the artist's work emanating from the desire that is curiosity. Whether understood as a developmental achievement, one related to the assumption of autonomy (to separation-individuation as psychoanalytically conceived by Margaret Mahler), or as a phylogenetic necessity, as neuroscientifically viewed by Panksepp, curiosity/SEEKING is a drive that stimulates imagination. Insofar as curiosity, creativity, and crisis (in Friston's sense of the homeostatic imperative that is the minimization of free energy) coalesce in imagination, however, in imagining the future as based upon models constructed from the past, it is this that behooves us to consider the philosophically (phenomenologically) expanded meaning of "image" itself.

Imagination is the capacity to produce mental "images," whether expressed conceptually or aesthetically, through the conjoining of information (garnered cognitively or through the senses) with one's inner world. In other words, as discussed earlier, *it is a process emanating from curiosity and leading to creativity.* But, once again, what is an image? Just what is this principal component of the imagination? Phenomenologically speaking, an image – whether two- or three-dimensional, whether rendered manually or digitally, whether aesthetically or cognitively expressed or existing solely in the mind – is generally considered reproductive. From the art historian to the neuroscientist, it is the representative function of the image, the image as re-presentation, that has long been assumed to define its essence. Yet it is this minimizing view of the symbolic power of the image, this consideration of its capacity (in conjunction with its etymology) to re-present what exists outside it, that accounts for the disregard of that which is inherent within all creative work (whatever the genre): the non-referential dimension of the image.

In its non-referential mode, which is to say its non-illusory, non-identifying means of exposing an inner affective state or some ambiguous quality of the external world, the abstract image reveals the tension and release intrinsic to the creative process itself. How related this may be to primary and secondary process mentation and/or to unconscious and conscious cognition implicates both the biology and the psychology of the MindBrain. Implicating the mobilization of what, in a somewhat different context, Rose terms "deeper emotional resonances from the past," art, like maternal attunement and infantile responsiveness, "provides a holding presence of reliably balanced tension and release."[81] And, in so doing, the work of art – whether visual or aural and, I would add, abstract art in particular – reveals the meaning of aesthetic resonance, the empirical meaning of the encounter with art. When the communication of feeling is differentiated from its generation in the viewer, the psychodynamic interplay at the core of aesthetic experience bears resemblance to the dyadic relation of psychoanalysis as well. Intersubjective? Empathic? Not in the sense implied by the notion of embodied simulation, but in the "neuropsychoaesthetic" sense to which the notion of "affective perception" (Rose's term) gives meaning.

"Neuropsychoaesthetics"

Neuroaesthetics and psychoaesthetics are rapidly gaining ground in the writing on the experience of art. However unwieldly, the term "neuropsychoaesthetics" might well enter the vocabulary of those considering what transpires in art's creation and reception, for the neurological and psychological are fundamentally inseparable as Freud knew from the start of his career in neuroscience prior to his founding of psychoanalysis. The attribution of meaning to a work of art was addressed by him most significantly in his 1910 work on Leonardo da Vinci, but I will return to the matter of psychobiography in the following chapter. The point I wish to make here is simply that curiosity, creativity, and the avoidance of crisis – as construed by Solms in neuropsychoanalysis and grounded in his research as well as that of Panksepp and Friston, and as applied to neuroaesthetics – are as much about the making of self as the making of art and about the interaction between them. "Self-making" – the "forward pull," the "becoming of mind" with which this book began – is life-long and reliant upon curiosity, upon the creativity and imagination ensuing from within it, and driven by crisis, whether that to which all are existentially vulnerable as individuals or ethically vulnerable as world citizens. Imagination can take form in aesthetics or manifest as an "ethical passion" (as Jardine calls it) when there is deep concern about a "world where there is no room for vulnerability, a world where everyone is becoming so commodified, mechanized, and programmed that they are never present to themselves."[82] In as much as psychoanalysis, for Kristeva, is a humanism (how not to concur with that assessment by Jardine?[83]) and in as much as Kristeva is a psychoanalyst strongly defensive of "the interpretive and creative process at the heart of global interdisciplinarity,"[84] one turns to her thinking, as one turned to that of Sartre, to that of Husserl, and that of the many philosophers and public intellectuals over time who questioned the critical diminution of humanistic values, of humanistic education, of humanism itself. One questions the meaning of freedom; one questions the "risk of thinking" (Jardine's term) and focuses on the interdisciplinarity of the neural mechanisms of the unconscious and consciousness at the core of psychoanalysis and neuroscience. As Jardine has written,

> In examining [the] sublimation of fear through artistic representation, Kristeva postulates [...] that the representation of violence can prevent violence in reality. That is, by refusing to erase what makes us fearful and violent, by finding a way to articulate and represent it, we avoid acting it out in real life. In this sense, representation functions in the same way as analysis does. By avoiding repression and embracing sublimation, representation can compensate for our loss of the loving maternal face and even accumulate joy through creativity. In the end, with any luck, the creative representation can circulate in the world as a singular active revolt – sometimes for centuries.[85]

In this context, the phenomenology of aesthetics comes to light and words like those by Samuel Beckett, in this case about James Joyce's *Work in Progress*, are given new meaning: "Here form *is* content, content *is* form," said Beckett. And these as well: "His writing is not *about* something; *it is that something itself*."[86]

Notes

1 The Adolph and Esther Gottlieb Foundation Archives, New York. https://www.gottliebfoundation.org/blog/2021/9/28/from-the-archives-the-jewell-letters-theres-no-such-thing-as-good-painting-about-nothing?format=amp
2 See Robert J. Zatorre and Valorie N. Salimpoor, "Why Music Makes Our Brain Sing," *The New York Times* (June 7, 2013). https://www.nytimes.com/2013/06/09/opinion/sunday/why-music-makes-our-brain-sing.html
3 See Zatoore and Salimpoor, "Why Music Makes Our Brain Sing."
4 Vittorio Gallese, "Aesthetics and the Unconscious: Toward an Embodied Neuroscience of the Image," JAPA, December 4, 2025. DOI: 10.1177/00030651251394305.
5 Valerie Hellstein, "De Kooning's Embodied Vision and Abstract Expressionism in the 1960s," in **Women Singing II* 1966 by Willem de Kooning*, Tate Research Publication, 2017. https://www.tate.org.uk/research/in-focus/women-singing-ii/de-koonings-embodied-vision
6 Sigmund Freud, "The Ego and The Id," in *Standard Edition*, vol. 19, 25.
7 Gilbert J. Rose, *Necessary Illusion: Art as Witness* (International Universities Press, Inc., 1996), 106.
8 Re these two phenomena, see Rose, *Necessary Illusion: Art as Witness*, 105–6.
9 Hellstein, "De Kooning's Embodied Vision and Abstract Expressionism in the 1960s."
10 Gallese, "Aesthetics and the Unconscious."
11 Gallese, "Aesthetics and the Unconscious."
12 Gallese, "Aesthetics and the Unconscious."
13 Andy Clark, *Surfing Uncertainty: Prediction, Action and the Embodied Mind* (Oxford University Press, 2016), 152.
14 Sigmund Freud, "Creative Writers and Day Dreaming," *Standard Edition*, vol. 9, 148.
15 Qtd. by Emet Brulin, "Gilles Deleuze's Unpublished Theory of Painting," *Nordic Art Review* (November 6, 2023). https://kunstkritikk.com/gilles-deleuzes-unpublished-theory-of-painting/#:~:text=Deleuze%20thus%20rejects%20the%20idea,a%20code%20for%20the%20future.%E2%80%9D
16 Cf., René de Ceccatty, "Le regard, le ciel et la mer," *Geneviève Asse. Galerie Antoine Laurentin* (2019), 15.

17 Samuel Beckett, "Geer van Velde," in *Disjecta*, ed. Ruby Cohn (Grove Press, 1984), 117.
18 Mark Solms, "Revision of Drive Theory," *JAPA* 69, no. 6 (2022): 1033.
19 Samuel Beckett, "Peintres de l'Empêchement" (1948), in *Disjecta*, ed. Ruby Cohn (Grove Press, 1984), 135.
20 Jacques Garelli, "Foreword: *Introduction to the Problematic of Gilbert Simondon*," in Gilbert Simondon, *Individuation in Light of Notions of Form and Information*, trans. Taylor Adkins (University of Minnesota Press, 2005/2020), xv–xvi.
21 Garelli, "Foreword: *Introduction to the Problematic of Gilbert Simondon*," xx.
22 Samuel Beckett, "Dante … Bruno. Vico. Joyce" (1929), in *Disjecta*, ed. Ruby Cohn (Grove Books, 1984), 22.
23 Doris Hering, "New London: Tenth Summer," *Dance Magazine* (Oct. 1957): 29.
24 Eliane Escoubas, "Maldiney – La peinture et le rythme," Séminaire Maldiney – ENS Philmaster – 8 novembre 2014 (trans. mine). https://www.henri-maldiney.org/sites/default/files/imce/hm.peinture_et_rythme.pdf
25 Maurice Merleau-Ponty, "Eye and Mind," in *The Primacy of Perception*, ed. James M. Edie (Northwestern University Press, 1964), 162.
26 See Jacques Garelli, *Rythmes et mondes: au revers de l'identité et de l'altérité* (Jérôme Million, 1993), chap. 4.
27 Garelli, "Foreword: *Introduction to the Problematic of Gilbert Simondon*," xvii, xxiii.
28 Garelli, "Foreword: *Introduction to the Problematic of Gilbert Simondon*," xxiii.
29 Garelli, "Foreword: *Introduction to the Problematic of Gilbert Simondon*," xx.
30 Garelli, "Foreword: *Introduction to the Problematic of Gilbert Simondon*," xxv.
31 Bruno Clément, *Henri Bergson, Prix Nobel de littérature* (Verdier, 2021), 101, 100, 101–2 (trans. mine).
32 Shaun Gallagher, "Precis: Enactivist Interventions," *Philosophical Studies* 176 (2019): 803–6. doi:10.1007/s11098-018-01230-8
33 Sigmund Freud, New Introductory Lectures, Lecture XXXI, "The Dissection of the Psychical Personality," *Standard Edition*, vol. 22, 79.
34 Personal communication.
35 Agnes Martin, *Writings*, ed. Dieter Schwarz (Edition Cantz). https://archive.org/stream/AgnesMartinWritings/Agnes%20Martin%20-%20Writings%20-%20Agnes%20Martin_djvu.txt
36 Merleau-Ponty, "Eye and Mind," in *The Primacy of Perception*, 123. Qtd. in Ludovica Lumer and Lois Oppenheim, *For Want of Ambiguity* (Bloomsbury Academic, 2019), 130.
37 Agnes Martin, qtd. in Dieter Schwarz, Preface, in Agnes Martin, *Writings*. https://dn790003.ca.archive.org/0/items/AgnesMartinWritings/Agnes%20Martin%20-%20Writings%20-%20Agnes%20Martin.pdf
38 Daniel M. Wegner, "The Mind's Self-Portrait," in *The Self from Soul to Brain*, ed. Joseph LeDoux, Jacek Debiec, and Henry Moss (The New York Academy of Sciences, 2003), 212.
39 Agnes Martin, lecture, "Beauty is the Mystery of Life." https://www.artbook.com/blog-excerpt-agnes-martin-beauty-is-the-mystery-of-life.html.
40 Suzan Campbell, Interview with Agnes Martin, May 15, 1989, Transcript, Archives of American Art, Smithsonian Institution, Washington, D.C., 17. Qtd. by Nancy Princenthal, *Agnes Martin: Her Life and Art* (Thames & Hudson, 2015), 93.
41 Qtd. by Princenthal, *Agnes Martin: Her Life and Art*, 131–32.
42 Martin, "Beauty is the Mystery of Life."
43 Arne Glimcher, *Agnes Martin: Paintings, Writings, Remembrances* (Phaidon, 2012), 13.
44 Mark Stevens, "Thin Gray Line," *Vanity Fair* (March 1989): 51. Qtd. by Princenthal, *Agnes Martin: Her Life and Art*, 206.

45 Shaun Gallagher, "The Unaffordable and the Sublime," *Continental Philosophical Review* 55 (2022): 431–45. doi:10.1007/s11007-022-09567-y. (Emphasis added.)
46 Sigmund Freud, "Civilization and Its Discontents," *Standard Edition*, vol. 21, 68, 72.
47 Jacques Garelli, *La gravitation poétique* (Mercure de France, 1966), 10 (trans. mine).
48 Beckett, "Peintres de l'Empêchement," 135.
49 Samuel Beckett, Letter to Axel Kaun (1937), in *Disjecta*, ed. Ruby Cohn (Grove Press, 1984), 172.
50 Beckett, Letter to Axel Kaun, 173.
51 See Lois Oppenheim, *The Painted Word: Samuel Beckett's Dialogue with Art* (The University of Michigan Press, 2000), 48.
52 Samuel Beckett, *Worstward Ho* (1983), in *NOHOW ON* (Calder Publications, 1992), 123.
53 Samuel Beckett, *Company* (1980), in *NOHOW ON* (Calder Publications, 1992), 18.
54 Beckett, *Worstward Ho*, 101.
55 Samuel Beckett, "What is the Word" (1989) (Faber and Faber, 2012), 228.
56 Laura Salisbury, "'What Is the Word': Beckett's Aphasic Modernism," *Journal of Beckett Studies* 17, no. 1–2 (2009): 78–126.
57 Salisbury, "'What Is the Word': Beckett's Aphasic Modernism."
58 Maurice Merleau-Ponty, "Eye and Mind" (1961), in *The Merleau-Ponty Aesthetics Reader: Philosophy and Painting* (Northwestern University Press, 1993), 122.
59 Enoch Brater, *The Drama in the Text: Beckett's Late Fiction* (Oxford University Press, 1994), 172–73.
60 Sigmund Freud, "The Unconscious" (Appendix C, Words and Things,), *Standard Edition*, vol. 14, 213–14.
61 Samuel Beckett to Lawrence Harvey, qtd. by Michael Coffey, *Beckett is Closed* (Foxrock Books, 2018), 41.
62 Ladislav Kesner, "The Predictive Mind and the Experience of Visual Art Work," *Frontiers in Psychology* 5 (2014). doi: 10.3389/fpsyg.2014.01417
63 Thomas Ogden, *The Primitive Edge of Experience* (Jason Aronson, Inc., 1989), 4.
64 Ogden, *The Primitive Edge of Experience*, 67.
65 Ogden, *The Primitive Edge of Experience*, 54.
66 Ogden, *The Primitive Edge of Experience*, 67, 71.
67 Thomas Ogden, "Ontological Psychoanalysis or 'What Do You Want To Be When You Grow Up?'" *The Psychoanalytic Quarterly* 88, no. 4 (2019): 664.
68 Ogden, "Ontological Psychoanalysis or 'What Do You Want To Be When You Grow Up?,'" 667.
69 Sigmund Freud, *New Introductory Lectures on Psychoanalysis: The Dissection of the Psychical Personality, Standard Edition*, vol. 22, 80.
70 Ogden, "Ontological Psychoanalysis or 'What Do You Want To Be When You Grow Up?,'" 667.
71 Jules Kerman, review of Thomas H. Ogden, *Coming to Life in the Consulting Room: Toward a New Analytic Sensibility, JAPA* 72, no. 2 (2024): 346, 349.
72 Rose, *Necessary Illusion: Art as Witness*, 111, 112–113.
73 Rose, *Necessary Illusion: Art as Witness*, 27, 112.
74 Lynn Gamwell and Mark Solms, *From Neurology to Psychoanalysis: Sigmund Freud's Neurological Drawings and Diagrams of the Mind* (Binghamton University Art Museum, State University of New York, 2006), 130.
75 Gamwell and Solms, *From Neurology to Psychoanalysis*, 91.
76 Freud, "Aphasie," in *A Moment of Transition: Two Neuroscientific Articles by Sigmund Freud*, trans. and ed. Mark Solms and Michael Saling (The Institute of Psycho-Analysis and Karnac Books, 1990), 32 (emphasis added).
77 Freud, "Aphasie," 145.

78 Freud, "Aphasie," 117 (emphasis added).
79 Jaak Panksepp, "Emotional Foundations of Creativity: The Brain's SEEKING System," in *Secrets of Creativity: What Neuroscience, the Arts, and Our Minds Reveal*, ed. Suzanne Nalbantian and Paul M. Matthews (Oxford Academic, 2019), 213.
80 Panksepp, "Emotional Foundations of Creativity," 216, 215.
81 Gilbert J. Rose, *Between Couch and Piano: Psychoanalysis, Music, Art and Neuroscience* (Brunner Routledge, 2004), 53.
82 Alice Jardine, *At the Risk of Thinking* (Bloomsbury Academic, 2020), 16.
83 See Jardine, *At the Risk of Thinking*, 245.
84 Jardine, *At the Risk of Thinking*, 15.
85 Jardine, *At the Risk of Thinking*, 229.
86 Beckett, "Dante . . . Bruno . Vico . . Joyce," 27.

Chapter 5

Post Postmodernism

From "Beyond 'Beyond...'" (Chapter Two) to "Post Postmodernism" (Chapter Five) via "...the Crisis of Uncertainty" and "The 'Imageless Image'" (Chapters Three and Four): Clearly, not only are the *empirical dimension of the aesthetic* and the *ontology of the subjectless artwork itself* at play (or PLAY) with one another in this book but the detachment of meaning from its indicator, the signified from the signifier, would appear to be as well. Or so the (post?) structuralist might say. Abstraction from or exclusion of the "real," the identifiable characteristic of modernist movements, preceded the deferral of meaning known as "différance," the uncertainty of language or semantic deconstruction that Jacques Derrida brought to the fore. In the era of the Derridean postmodern, the variability of meaning left behind the presence of what, however abstractly, was referenced by the modernist. The variability of meaning transcended in ambiguity the rendering of absence as present, the rendering owed previously to abstraction in painting, absurdist playwriting, and much poetry both in the United States and abroad. Yet, in PLAY, and in the SEEKING that creatively promotes it, in the two emotional drive systems accounting for aesthetic experience, the modern and postmodern may be said to be deeply conjoined.

The relation of modernism to the postmodern has already been the subject of a great many writings and is not my focus here. On the contrary: My concern is with that for which the modernist/postmodernist debate cannot account: The potential relation of the ahistorical to the crises (the anti-humanitarian world crises, the anti-humanistic direction of artificial intelligence, the anti-humanities direction of higher education and the deflation of higher education altogether) with which we now contend. But the claim by the literary critic Marjorie Perloff that "we have always been modern"[1] as countered by the philosopher of science Bruno Latour, author of *We Have Never Been Modern*, is noteworthy in the present context for the following reason: As we have seen, the homeostatic crisis continually averted by the minimization of uncertainty ("Friston's Law") and the modern-postmodern chaos (Beckett's "mess") in which visual,

DOI: 10.4324/9781003566755-6

literary, theatrical, and musical artists find both relief and "joy" oblige one to consider "the role of surprisal in aesthetic experience." Yet the conflict of perspective – of visual processing, embodied simulation, and neuropsychoanalysis – on the experience in question inhibits our grasp of that very role. The phenomenology of Merleau-Ponty, like that of Maldiney, Simondon, and Garelli whose work reveals his profound influence, affords, by way of the focus on the ontological, greater understanding of the integrative value of each of these perspectives. This is to say that it affords greater understanding of aesthetic experience in and of itself, greater understanding of just what it is: namely, *a multi-determined, fundamentally inquisitory and creative energic engagement offering pleasure by way of the sensory, by way of perception, and nourished by unconscious and conscious association and their affective constitution.*

"Neuropsychoaesthetics" Redux

"When the sense is sleep, the words go to sleep. [...] When the sense is dancing, the words dance." So said Beckett of Joyce, whose *Work in Progress* was not simply to be read, Beckett deemed, but "looked at and listened to."[2] We look once again at the painting by David Smith, a painting that dances, that is not only to be viewed but watched – *and sensed.* It entices a prolonged viewing (a watching) precisely because, as we look, we sense the movement of the lines. Rather than the gesture of the artist, rather than a simulation, what is corporally experienced is a perceptual sensing of the movement constituting the painting itself. It is not because there is movement depicted by the artist (though there is), but because the painting puts in high relief the aesthetic experience. "Here form *is* content, content *is* form," we recall Beckett's having written of Joyce demonstrating not empathy, not intersubjectivity, but the actuality of the aesthetic encounter.

The "neuropsychoaesthetic" point of view is meant to account for the corporeal dimension (neither solely ocular nor motorically simulative), along with the free energy perspective of Friston (minus the conclusions drawn by some), into the neuropsychoanalytic foundation explicated by Solms. This results in a way of thinking about the experience of art that accounts for the complex ways in which the mind and body function relationally, in which the MindBrain functions unilaterally (even if its structuring calls for a bilateral, which is to say a subjective and objective or dual-monist, consideration), a way of thinking that echoes the work of yet another French philosopher and literary critic: Maurice Blanchot.

Most notably and most relevant to my purpose here are Blanchot's ideas of "disaster" and "detachment," ideas both Derridean (post-structuralist) and not. Consider the following passages excerpted from Blanchot's *The Writing of the Disaster*:

> The disaster, unexperienced. It is what escapes the very possibility of experience – it is the limit of writing. This must be repeated: the disaster of de-scribes. Which does not mean that the disaster, as the force of writing, is excluded from it, it is beyond the pale of writing or extratextual.
>
> Reading is anguish, and this is because any text, however important, or amusing, or interesting it may be (and the more engaging it seems to be), is empty – at bottom it doesn't exist; you have to cross an abyss, and if you do not jump, you do not comprehend.
>
> Beyond seriousness there is play, but beyond play, and seeking that which out-plays (the way the disaster de-scribes), there is the gratuitous, from which no escape. It is what by chance befalls, and I fall beneath it, having always fallen already. Days and nights go by in silence. Such as the word.[3]

How stunning the confluence of principles and tropes: "Disaster" – crisis, uncertainty, the chaos of "de-scribes"; the emptiness of the text that "at bottom [...] doesn't exist" – "artworks are actually as dead as doornails" (Solms), art is "a little bit of nothing" (Rivers); the "abyss" to be crossed, the "jump" required to comprehend; the play, the "seeking that which out-plays" (Panksepp). How stunning the confluence of two of Blanchot's often-repeated concepts with the art we have been considering: First, the notion of "*il y a*" (the "there is") – describable in terms of anonymity, the "state which precedes all meaning," to cite Joseph Kuzma[4] – stunningly confluent not only with the ambiguity, but the immateriality projected in the painting of John Day, Geneviève Asse, and Agnes Martin, among many others. And stunningly confluent, as well, with "the presence of the absence" so recurrent in Beckett, confluent with the ontology of art that remains without a subject yet is as pervasively impervious to nullification as it is resistant to empathic intrusion. Second, the concept of "the neuter" in Blanchot, a notion having nothing to do with gender, but which Kuzma eloquently describes as "a word's ability to suspend and remark itself in such a way that it ceases to signify what it signifies, and it begins to drift into the indeterminacy of multiple meanings," a notion striking in its similarity with Derridean *différance* in as much as it "exposes every word to an infinity of meanings, making language possible on the condition that it is constantly traversed by a radical alterity that both precedes and exceeds it." In establishing "the non-coincidence of language with itself,"[5] "the neuter" is profoundly Beckettian ("what is the word"). And in its effort to find meaning where there isn't any, it is so as well ("make sense who may").

But leaving this philosopher of the literary, this theoretician of the modern and postmodern, at the intersection between them, I return briefly to their defining characteristics in the interest of engaging with what may constitute their aftermath. However much associated with minimalism, the oceanic, or the sublime, however much *dis*associated from the representational and the innately personal, abstract painting (whether that of Martin, Rothko, Day, Gottlieb, or Asse, whether that of any other painter of the un- or minimally identifiable), like absurdist theater (that, for example, of Beckett), is *modernist* in the sense that it implies experimentation and abstraction. The word "abstract" in painting relates, of course, to the idea of using color and form to render visual the experiential; specifically, the experience of a non-objectifiable world. One might, once again, be inclined to describe it as a manner of removing (abstracting) from within the world particulars whose deformation offers pleasure, however the source of that pleasure (kinesthetic or other) may be defined. One might be inclined to describe it, as I have also done, in terms of the presencing through absence (the "imageless image") and the play (PLAY) with form.

Postmodernism was defined in the latter half of the twentieth century by the formalist views of structuralism and post-structuralism. With regard to the former, Claude Lévi-Strauss comes first to mind for his application of its premises to anthropology, its application of what Ferdinand de Saussure, the Swiss linguist, had brought to light: the value of semiological systems. Regarding the latter, Jacques Derrida, Michel Foucault, Julia Kristeva, and Roland Barthes are most easily associated with that perspective (although not all accepted the classification). Beginning in the 1960s, post-structuralism called into question the idea of inherent structures upon whose underlying relations the attribution of meaning was dependent. A reaction against the premises of structuralism, post-structuralism rejected the certainty of such relations (whether binary oppositions or similarities) and focused on deconstructing the idea of fixed, non-experience-related meanings. Many are those who have written on the subject of the postmodern, some within the context of history, which is to say within the context of cultural change, the transition away from the modern to whatever the postmodern was understood to mean, and some within the context of aesthetic theory. Whereas the modern was viewed as a reaction against tradition, the postmodern was explored by the aesthetician as something beyond that negative response. But then, as already noted, there are those who would argue that we have never been modern or that we will always be modern, doing away with the postmodern altogether. However much postmodernism was the subject of late twentieth-century Western philosophical and critical writing, in sum, there are those who profess that humankind has never been modern and those who profess that it has always been nothing but. Yet what do we really mean by "modern"? And what does someone, like Bruno Latour, mean when they say we have never been modern? Or someone like Marjorie Perloff mean when they say we will always be modern?

The term "modernism" was used by the critic of literary modernism Daniel Albright to contradict the notion that "there is no such thing as a school of artists," that "an idea such as *influence* among artists arises from sheer

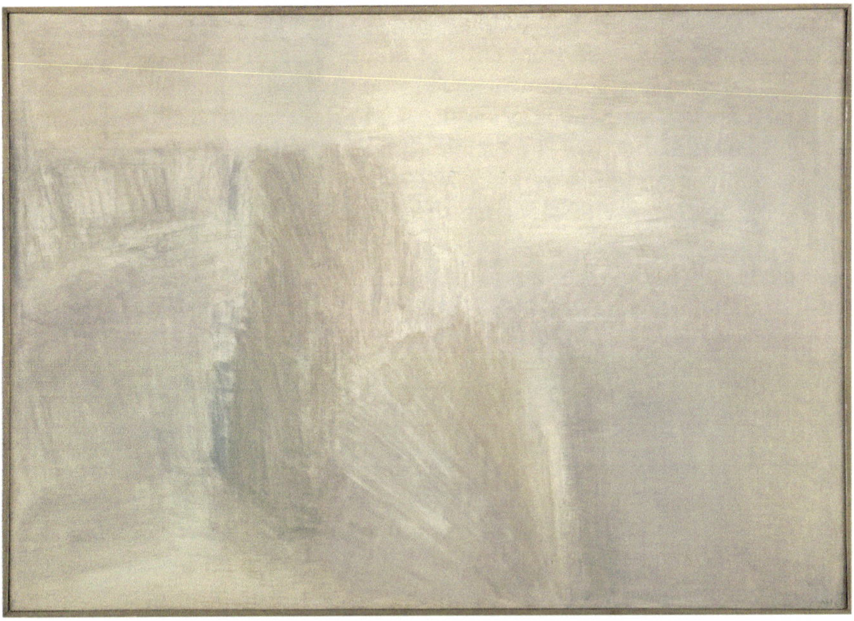

Figure 5.1 Geneviève Asse (1923–2021), Amsterdam – 1965. Oil on canvas. Collection musée des beaux-arts, La Cohue © Musées de Vannes.

intellectual laziness." This is an argument that contradicts, he noted, the "intuition that certain works of art look like one another; that, among many works of art produced at the same time or in the same place, there are family resemblances."[6] A definition of the modernist era in the arts that would account for such resemblances is offered by Albright as follows:

> [M]odernism is a testing of the limits of aesthetic construction. According to this perspective, the modernists tried to find the ultimate bounds of certain artistic possibilities: volatility of emotion (expressionism); stability and inexpressiveness (the new objectivity); accuracy of representation (hyperrealism); absence of representation (abstractionism); purity of form (neoclassicism); formless energy neo barbarism; cultivation of the technological present (futurism); cultivation of the prehistoric past (the mythic method). [...] Much of the strangeness, the stridency, the exhilaration of modernist art can be explained by this strong thrust toward the verges of the aesthetic experience: after the 19th century had established a remarkably safe, intimate center where the artist and the audience could dwell, the twentieth century reaches out to the freakish circumferences of art.[7]

Yet this is but a single interpretation of the modernist endeavor, Albright concedes, and just as there exist many modernisms, the temporal delimitations vary. But more to the point, we encounter once again, this time in the context of artistic frontiers, the notion of crisis: "Modernist art has existed in an almost continual state of crisis concerning the boundaries between one art medium and another," Albright contends. "Is a painting worth 1000 words, or is it impossible to find verbal equivalent of an image, even if millions of words were used? Are music and literature two different things, or two aspects of the same thing? This is a question confronted by artists of every age but the artists of the modernist period found a special urgency here." In fact, "some artists tried to erase the boundaries among music and literature and the visual arts, while other artists tried to build foot-thick walls."[8]

Why Does It Matter?

Once again, we ask why it matters. Why does it matter if there was or was not a "special urgency" to the modernist artistic endeavor? Why does it matter if there was or was not "an almost continual state of crisis" regarding the boundaries of artistic mediums? Why, what's more, does it matter if we have always or never been modern? And, in conjunction with these questions, why, we might ask, did literary and visual artists over a half century ago, became focused on the social implications of their work? What kind of cultural (or possibly even political) change did they anticipate their art might reflect or even inspire? Was Sartre's central notion of freedom and the responsibility, given that freedom, to choose (with not doing so reflecting a choice in itself) uniquely modern? "Un cri de douleur est signe de la douleur qui le provoque. Mais un chant de douleur est à la fois la douleur elle-même et autre chose que la douleur" ("A cry of pain is a sign of the pain that provokes it. But a song of pain is at once the pain itself and something other than the pain"), as noted earlier, was what he famously stated in his 1948 work *Qu'est-ce que la littérature?*.[9] Was this expression of the inherent duality of art an anticipation of the postmodern? Was Kristeva's recognition of "the need to think and rethink 'freedom,'" to differentiate the freedom that follows adaptation to what is external to oneself from the freedom of "eternal questioning," of curiosity, as "a way of being in the world," to cite Alice Jardine, uniquely postmodern?[10] Was Kristeva's recognition postmodern before it was modern? Was the recognition by Sartre and Kristeva of the relation between art and the mind, not in the surrealist sense of art's expression of the unconscious, but in the psychoanalytic sense of the value of sublimation, more post than pre? We ask why it matters and we ask in conjunction with that question why one Western society, one cultural milieu, is more attentive to the aesthetic revolutions or pronouncements of the intellectual than another. Which are they, when do they respond as they do, and why?

It matters because the modernist aesthetic posed essential questions: How much is possible in art and how does art relate to perception as intertwined with the psyche? What is art without the spectator, listener, or reader's subjective experience? Is art ontically significant or only ontologically so? The postmodern aesthetic posed others: Some questions concerning language (its expressivity or lack of); some concerning identity and the ego-world relation (with the questions of agency, self-reflexivity, *mise en abyme*, and *différance* not far behind[11]); all related to the uncertainty of meaning with its diversity of origins. *Both unveiled the crisis of uncertainty, the crisis of the fluidity of meaning*. We find this undeniably in Beckett, a literary and theatrical artist whose fragmented poetry, novels, and theatrical pieces – which is to say whose play (PLAY) with the short-circuiting of all – appear modeled on the sensory perspective of the eye while the visual prototype, in allowing his art to be, is precisely what subverts it. Causing the "absurd" to take on an additional layer of meaning, an aesthetic layer lying over and above the existential, it is this that causes failure to be a persistent threat. In a sense, Beckett's fragmentation and reductionism confirm the conjecture – derived from Hegel and demonstrable, via Duchamp and Warhol – that art has reached an end. Not the end of stoppage, but the end signified by those who write of the perpetuation of the making of art beyond the completion of art's history. The end of Beckett's writing, to which the shorter prose, in particular, so distinctly calls attention, refers not to the putting down of the pen, but to the kind of writing that took place in response to its own self-consciousness. Simultaneously, however, Beckett's reductionism confirms that, insofar as his is a totalizing art (a synthesis of sight and sound, poetry and drama, literature and choreography), within its very minimalism a concrete universal is revived. What lies beyond the fragmentation, in other words, is *an ontology of art for which the modernist/postmodernist debate cannot account*. We would do well, therefore, to maintain with regard to his work, as to that of the painters intermittently discussed throughout this book as well, a low modernist view of the high modernist distinction between the late modernist and postmodernist aesthetic, or so one might, with more than a touch of irony, conclude.

It matters because we are foreseeing crisis, on the edge of crisis, in the midst of crisis: Humanitarian crisis, cultural crisis, identity crisis, climate crisis, social crisis ensuing from the rapid transformation of artificial intelligence, the unmooring of collective values, and more. And all are about uncertainty, about feeling, about care (or CARE). "Music is a powerful inducer of feelings," Antonio Damasio has written. And the "emotivity" associated with "certain instrumental sounds, modes, keys, and compositions" is "comparable to the emotivity found for colors, shapes" and more. So, too, the movement of dance. "The case for the homeostatic function of the visual arts – which begin with cave paintings – and for the traditional oral storytelling in poetry, theater, and political exhortation, is not difficult to make," Damasio claims.[12] And it is this homeostatic function – this uncertainty, the necessity that is prediction, and the correction of prediction error – as I have stressed, that drives our curiosity (SEEKING), our need to reduce tension through play (PLAY), and thereby our creativity as well.

It matters because, in response to Damasio's well-formulated question "Is There a Biology behind the Cultural Crisis?," it would appear there is.[13] And "understanding" (a term to be *understood*, as Niels Bohr reminded us) the biological bedrock of culture, while not providing the entire answer, aids us in coping with the challenge that is the crisis defining of the human condition. It aids us in coping with uncertainty and allows for appreciation of the curiosity and creativity impelled by that uncertainty. This is to say that it matters because the dynamics of aesthetic experience are akin to how individuals and cultures alike cope with dysregulation, and "understanding" the nature of that experience can only enrich the satisfaction and pleasure, the regulatory functions, associated with all human experience.

It matters because "understanding" – the foundation, after all, of neuroaesthetics and psychoanalysis – allows us to know why knowing matters, to know how it relates to experience, and what the meaning of experience is. It matters because it is "art's lifesaving power to harness vital rhythm to aesthetic form" that "salvage[s] a rudimentary self from total chaos," as Gilbert Rose has said. While art cannot necessarily steady an ego in distress, as he puts it, it can be framed by the protection against uncertainty to which the Free Energy Principle attests insofar as early-life "symbiotic modes of relating inner and outer do not atrophy," do not yield to something other than what they are from the beginning of life. "Rather," as he explains, "they undergo continuing development and differentiation." They both protect and enrich. And it is the interplay of these relational modes with the self and object representations that become increasingly demarcated over time that contributes to the "richness of life – including, especially, art and the creative process."[14]

It matters because in the frame of both the modern and postmodern – whether the lineage from one to the other or the schism between them – it is both *the meaning of experience* and *the defeat of determinism* that unfold. My alignment with Solms' perspective on the role of surprisal in aesthetic experience, as with the absence of empathy in the "as-dead-as-doornails" work of art and with "Friston's Law" as well as Beckett's "mess," calls into question our understanding of "embodiment," the buzzword in multiple areas of inquiry today. Indeed, challenging, as in the preceding chapter, the notion of embodied simulation (understood to be the motoric objectivation of empathic resonance) requires questioning the phenomenon of embodiment itself independent of the multiple other phenomena with which it is increasingly conjoined. The embodiment of transference in the psychoanalytic dyad, the embodiment of cognition in the concept of mind, the embodiment of AI in the robot and related physical entities, and so on: what does it really mean? While not defined culturally, not limited to the distinctiveness of any particular group, it is unidentified with the human "body" (except with regard to aging and the passage of time), with that which connotes the physical entity belonging to a single human being. Aural, visual, tactile embodiment: Each can be simulated insofar as it is universally experienced. Like the mind, the body, moreover, is a process of becoming (as opposed to being fixed from the start of life) and it "constitutes a prior dimension of experience that is universally shared among all subjects and the world they inhabit," as Jason Baskin has written. Thus it is "social or collective, rather than individual." "[W]hen Merleau-Ponty talks about embodied subjectivity," Baskin further explains, "he refers neither to an individual 'I' nor a communal 'we,' neither an individual self nor a delimited group of individuals united by shared ideas, experiences or practices. Instead, he refers to a generalized, anonymous and universal 'one' [...] that precedes any individual self or articulated community."[15] This is an exceedingly important point in that it is this "universally shared" dimension of experience "in which we all participate as anonymous subjects of perception" that gives meaning to humanism. It gives meaning to a worldview associated with the Renaissance for its focus on the meaning and value of humanity, but which knows no chronology. Humankind is humankind. Yet humanism, linked with humanitarianism in its centering on the value of human life, choice, and culture – the former with an eye on the life of the self, the latter on that of the other – would appear to be temporal by virtue of the very lack of humanitarianism seemingly endemic to the state of the world at present. Considered as embodiment, however, whether in its symbolic, representational, abstract, rhythmic, or other components of form, art recenters experience to rejoin it to its atemporal and humanistic constituents. Mark Rothko "focused on the essences" in his work, "the defining elements of what it is to be human," Christopher Rothko has written. And, writing of his father's use of color in the artist's signature paintings, the sectionals, he notes that they are "the painted expression of what it is to be human and alive."[16]

It is when we consider art an extraction from the materiality of the bodily presence, a projection much like that described by Freud with regard to the ego ("the projection of a surface"), that we enter the realm of the chiasmic interplay that Merleau-Ponty described. We enter the realm of the "flesh of the world," as he called the ontological crossover of feeling and being felt, of perceiving and being perceived, that connects self and world. In this "flesh of the world" the body is not only a perceptible subject but a perceiving object and, like words, like brushstrokes, and musical notes, it is the abstraction from material presence in which the self and non-self are intertwined.

We see Merleau-Ponty's ontological perspective played out in Beckett, in the juxtaposition of the I and the "not I," in the "she" of Beckett's play where Mouth's pronominal refusal to accept the sentience of the subjective first-person is what constitutes the drama. What *Not I* reveals is an abstraction, and "uncanny," or Freud's *unheimlich* (the simultaneously familiar and unfamiliar), is perhaps what best describes its congruence not only with Merleau-Ponty's understanding of the fundamental role played by the body in the self's apprehension of its ontology, but with Solms' description of the experiential as well. Phenomenologically, neuroscientifically, and aesthetically, Beckett's work (*Not I* in particular, but several other of his other writings as well) reveals precisely what Solms terms "three levels of experience: (1) the affective or phenomenal level of the self as subject, a.k.a. first-person perspective; (2) the perceptual or representational level of the self as object, a.k.a. second-person perspective; (3) the abstracted or re-representational level of the self as object in relation to other objects, a.k.a. third-person perspective."[17]

Phenomenologically (Merleau-Ponty), aesthetically (Beckett), and neuroscientifically (Solms), we surpass the modern/postmodern dialectic when embodiment is viewed as encapsulating all three levels of experience. Mark Rothko, Adolph Gottlieb, Agnes Martin, Geneviève Asse: All strove to reveal the universality of experience through embodiment in color and form. As in Beckett's, we find a striving in their work to reveal the passion of creativity however threatened it may be. If it matters *not to conclude* whether we have always or never been modern *but to consider* the question, it is because it matters to "understand" *the drive to embody in the aesthetic the nature of experience*. It matters to "understand" the curiosity and reality testing (the SEEKING and PLAY) that drives the creative bypassing of crisis: "Ever tried. Ever failed. No matter. Try again. Fail again. Fail better," to cite once more Beckett's 1983 novella *Worstward Ho*. It matters to "understand," just as it does the biological necessity that is the formulation of prediction and the correction of prediction error, the reduction of uncertainty (free energy) aligned with the chaos of Beckett's "mess."

No less real than the brain for its immateriality, the mind is one's feeling self (as Solms often reminds us). This is confirmed by the very idea that aesthetic experience (that of viewer, reader, listener alike) exceeds the "intercorporeal resonance" (as Gallese terms it) of embodied simulation to include the resonance of art with the affect it stimulates as opposed to simulates. This arousal of emotion – incomparable to a *transmission* of affect (as in empathy) and consisting, rather, in its *incitement* – is conspicuously apprehended in the metaphysical abstractions of many modern artists. It is this kindling of feeling that inspired the postmodernist to search the source, the Derridean "trace" signaling deferred associations, and what inspires us now to question, in this post postmodernist era, the neuroscience so deeply intertwined with the aesthetic as with the psychoanalytic.

The engagement of neuroscience with psychoanalysis allows for an understanding of the aesthetic beyond the objectivation of feeling. The art object, being no more an object than the feeling with which it resonates, is a dynamic entity cocreated with the artist by the beholder, listener, or reader. And it is this perceptually driven phenomenon that constitutes the activity we call aesthetic experience. How not to agree with Gallese's assertion that to understand aesthetic experience we must consider the encoding of movement in the image?[18] But that movement is far greater than the gestural, far more than the brushstroke pre-reflectively apprehended by the viewer; it even far exceeds the motoric apprehension by the listener of the rhythm to which one is impelled to dance. Gallese himself has extended of late his explanation of embodied simulation, his definition of the "temporal activation that is bodily in nature," as he defines it, to include a dimension he rightly assesses as "often overlooked in both philosophical aesthetics and neuroscientific accounts": the reactivation of "previous embodied schemata – motor, affective, mnemonic – imbued with a new salience." Writing of the visual image, he now qualifies it as the reconfiguration of "what was already latent in the subject's body," a process belonging to a wider conception of the Freudian unconscious than repression, one that is "temporal, embodied, and relational." The image, as he now explains it, "acts less as a representation to be decoded and more as an affective device that mobilizes sensorimotor and affective schemata – activating what could be called an embodied *mneme* of relational life."[19]

This is a valuable broadening of the concept for it underscores the psychobiology of perception that allows for greater understanding of aesthetic experience as neuroscientifically and psychoanalytically approachable. Rhythm (aural and visual), movement, color, shapes, words and their syntactical assembly require consideration from the unifying perspective of the neural construction of the sensorial and the ego-world relation; in other words, the interaction between them. Art and aesthetic experience, I would argue, cannot be comprehensively considered from either perspective alone, no more than from the "purely visualist paradigm," the "oculocentrism," that "in aesthetic theory and empirical aesthetics has privileged the eye as the primary organ of aesthetic access, while marginalizing the bodily and affective dimensions of perception," as Gallese has said.[20] In this post postmodernist era, when lived experience and our understanding of that experience is expanding due to an increased understanding of the science behind both the physicality and affectivity of the body, of the MindBrain that encodes through learning and memory what *was* experienced for its predictive value of what *will* be experienced, neither is to be privileged.

Psychobiographical Inquiry

In the context of neuropsychoanalysis, SEEKING and PLAY, to make the point yet once more, are the two emotional drive systems giving rise to creative expression. In so doing, they initiate ways of moving forward, of going on, of "becoming." SEEKING affords learning by way of curiosity and exploration; PLAY supports imaginative experimentation and creative expression as well as social interaction. Interrelated, these two emotional drive systems are phylogenetically and homeostatically necessary for the aversion of what is termed "crisis." Artistically, they contribute to the sublimation of what might otherwise be experienced as some sort of conflictual dysregulation, some sort of emotional distress ensuing from the discord between repressed desire and superego disallowance. Back in the day, rather than viewing sublimation as a healthy means of suspending if not resolving such conflict, there was a tendency to pathologize the artist. While we have moved away from that inclination, from that stereotype of the creative individual, it is not that we have given it up so much as found a means to cloud it. Psychobiography would appear to have something to offer when the subject in question has significantly impacted history broadly speaking. Presuming the availability of extensive material for research and sound knowledge of the socio-cultural milieu with which the subject is identified, such an offering, however, is not to be confused with the conceptualization of the psychodynamic components of artistic creativity or its reception, components primarily knowable only hypothetically and, even when able to be biographically validated, otherwise compromising.

"Perception per se is also a creative act," the late Austrian psychoanalyst and archivist of the Sigmund Freud Archives, Kurt Eissler, wisely reminded by letter a clinical colleague who, in discussing a paper he had written about Picasso, had remarked that he had been aiming for what he termed a "psychoanalytic iconography." In a previous conversation Eissler had been more critical of that colleague's psychobiographic analysis claiming that, while a very interesting paper, it failed to explain Picasso's creativity. In the letter in question, he explained his earlier comment by saying, "Externalization is not enough. In perception we externalize a retinal process." "Thinking about it I must admit that the existing iconography as met in the current histories of art should have to be rewritten when you apply a [psychoanalytic] viewpoint," he further, if somewhat ambiguously, commented. Phyllis Greenacre, also writing to Leon Hoffman, author of the Picasso paper entitled "Picasso and the Painter Model Theme: Multiple Identifications and Creative Transformations of Aggressive Conflicts," appeared similarly ambiguous (similarly hesitant?) about assigning, as fully as had Hoffman, aggression to Picasso's creativity: "I would only say that I think in some instances, it is especially the effort to transform, or even in a sense to assign especially those libidinized aggressive pressures in the service of art." And: "I have a further question whether the aggression is basically an obligatory pressure of special inborn growth needs."[21] Both Eissler and Greenberg were impressed by Hoffman's study of what he calls "the effect of the psychology of the artist on his art," his exploration of the painter's effort "to master some intense intrapsychic conflict" relating to his father while taking care "not to make broad interpretive leaps."[22] Indeed, Hoffman prudently recognizes the hypothesizing inherent in a psychobiographical explanation of art, in any attempt at revealing the unconscious fantasies of an artist. And he recognizes the unconscious identifying with the artist such a critical analysis might produce. Despite the avoidance of such "interpretive leaps" in this psychobiographical account of Picasso's imagery, however, the reader is left with the question that both Eissler and Greenberg, both highly notable psychoanalysts, appear to be raising: Just what is the effect of such explanation on one's viewing of Picasso's art?

I briefly considered "the role of surprisal in aesthetic experience" (Chapter 3) in the context of "consciousness as felt uncertainty" (as per Solms) and Friston's Free Energy Principle. There is, however, yet another way to regard surprisal in such experience and that, once again, is in terms of the philosophical or, more precisely, the phenomenological. The French philosopher Gaston Bachelard wrote of the ontological import of the image and the communion of the image maker with the observer. In noting the surprisal inherent in the creative act, inherent in the eruption of the imagination ontologically verifiable in its expression, Bachelard removes the psychology of the artist from the act of creation: "In all psychological research," he claimed, "we can, of course, bear in mind psychoanalytical methods for determining the personality of a poet, and thus find a measure of the pressures – but above all of the oppressions – that a poet has been subjected to in the course of his life. But the poetic act itself, the sudden image, *the flare-up of being in the imagination*, are inaccessible to such investigations."[23] In his phenomenological account of the imagination, the philosopher removes the focus of psychobiography as though in response to this very question.

It is in the context of drive energy, moreover – wherein the union of the structural with the dynamic, the objective with the subjective, the brain with the mind is indisputable, wherein the physiology of the one is manifested in the feeling of the other – that we understand why the psychohistorical cannot truly attain the validity to which it aspires. It is in this context, as we previously saw, that the "Becoming Mind" study with which I began and the Panksepp–Solms–Friston understanding of development as the reconciliation of drives with each other attain their exceptional degree of congruence. *For, in the sensorial experience of the infant and developing child – in whom the continuity of self and "becoming" of mind, in whom the integration or reconciliation of drive demands, are achieved through memory and learning, through prediction modeling and prediction error remediation – it is the energic forces of drive that constitute the "forward pull."* Irreducible to libidinal pleasure alone, to "libidinized aggressor pressures," as Greenberg put it, an historical trajectory is neuropsychoanalytically, if not psychobiographically, comprehensible. This is to say that there is a history to be traced but, over and above the question of its accuracy, whether that tracing can ultimately contribute in some significant way to one's experience of a work of art remains to be seen.

Psychobiography has a sullied reputation precisely because it tends to put the artist on the couch in search of a narrative informed by pathology. Insofar as aesthetic experience may be adversely impacted by assumptive knowledge of an artist's inner world, the danger intrinsic to psychobiography is its being all too often misguided for being primarily based on supposition. Indeed, examples of supposition presented as fact and such fact presented as justification for this or that attribution of meaning are far too readily available in the psychoanalytic literature devoted to art. What associations are offered? Where is the transference? This is not to say, of course, that nothing is to be learned from psychohistorical exploration, but that self-awareness in the process is essential.

Michael Coffey, author of *Beckett's Children: A Literary Memoir*, puts in high relief the value of such awareness. An adoptee himself, one forever preoccupied with the identity of his own biological parents, Coffey has long sought the truth regarding the possibility of Samuel Beckett's having fathered the American poet Susan Howe. Now known not to be true, at least according to Howe's claim that there is DNA evidence to the contrary, a claim that Coffey has stated he has no reason to disbelieve, that question is cast aside in favor of these: "[H]ow did it affect Susan Howe's evolving identity and practice as a writer to be in her fifties before discovering for sure who her father was?" And "if Susan was unsure for all that time, what was Beckett sure of, and how did the uncertainty, if he was not shielded from it, affect his work?"[24] Had Beckett been disturbed by the possibility that he had begotten a child, how could that not have entered into his writings, writings where both children (real or imagined) and uncertainty play prominent roles. Here is how Coffey replied when asked just why it was important to him to know:

> What meaning would it have for me (or us) if Beckett was aware of Susan Howe's uncertainty (of paternity)? (Think of *Godot*, which begins "Nothing to be done" and continues, "Nothing is certain when you are around," exchanges between our pseudocouple Didi and Gogo.) It might change how we view the unattended children that wander in and out of his works, often as messengers. We might consider this uncertainty as another element to his trauma that was channeled into the frenzy of writing just after the war that produced his central masterworks. It might reset or refresh the discussions about Beckett's relation to the body and the sexual act. Consider if he was aware of a young woman's torment across the Atlantic. We do know he was very sympathetic when faced with the struggles or sufferings of dear friends. [...] we might see the object (the texts, the subject) differently with this slight change in perspective.

Even more to the point, however, here is how that reply began:

> Being an adoptee, a literary person and a writer, I know that I am especially sensitive to the issue of literary inheritance. I spent many decades pursuing my identity through writing, through the lives of writers, through literature, looking for clues as to who I was and the evidence of my own practice and the manners of my reading. Whether I have discovered a sense of myself through this process or imagined it I cannot say. But I can say it is one, the other, or a mixture of both.[25]

The value of the psychohistorical is greatly enhanced by the self-awareness to which Coffey subscribes throughout this emotionally unsettling, poetically enticing, and exceedingly rich study of the literary subjects. While not limited to the psychobiographic as such, but deeply investigative of his own predilections as well as those of these authors, this work manifests just how exposure of the psychodynamic can enhance our understanding of the aesthetic. All too often, however, whether or not it is articulated, as in this example, the lack of self-awareness in the psychobiographical exploration results in the very kind of determinist perspective, the very kind of eventualizing, that both the modernist and postmodernist sought to reject. Evolutionary thinking, economic configurations, Newtonian physics: all bore the stamp of the determinism rejected by modernism in favor of relativity and the subjective; all bore the stamp of the determinism rejected by postmodernism in favor of a socio-historical contingency. So, too, the psychobiographical trajectory lacking in attentiveness to the unpredictability, the uncertainty of the encounter with art. "Tension, uncertainty and the violation of our expectations are part and parcel of good art; as has been noted since the earliest philosophical writings in aesthetics," Sander Van de Cruys, Jacopo Frascaroli, and Karl Friston have written. "Indeed, the genuine moments of discovery – that art enables – seem to demand tensions and uncertainties (change) as much as they demand closure and certainty (order)."[26] The timing of the aesthetic encounter, the mood of the beholder, and more play into the experience of art, as previously stressed, to deconstruct the determinism of the storyline informing the psychobiographically oriented critic's narrative.

If pathologizing the artist is no longer common today, a broader focus on object reparation and intrapsychic conflict being more frequent points of psychobiographical departure than the hasty stereotyping of yesterday, just how do we conceive of the relation of the truly pathological to art when known to exist or have existed? "I fight pain, anxiety, and fear every day, and the only method I have found that relieves my illness is to keep creating art," Japanese artist Yayoi Kusama famously wrote in her autobiography.[27] How she finds relief in her art is certainly of interest, as is her choosing to live in a psychiatric hospital and maintain a studio nearby. Why she succumbed to mental illness, what caused her panic attacks and hallucinations, is another question entirely. And that is a question that remains, for the museumgoer, unanswerable or at least irrelevant. What is *not* unanswerable, however, and what has bearing on our understanding of aesthetic experience is how the very knowledge of her struggle with mental illness impacts our viewing of her work.

Like Kusama, Agnes Martin, as is commonly known, suffered from schizophrenia. What does knowing about her psychosis do to our experience of her work? How much is the preoccupation with a kind of selflessness, the deep concern with the unrecognizable so evident in her art (a perspective attested to by her own prolific commentary on painting), impacted by her life story? Might our viewing experience be in some way enhanced by our knowledge of her mental illness or, conversely, might that knowledge constitute some sort of impediment to a deep resonance with it? Whether it be with regard to the strictly implemented grids – forms as obsessive in their conception as perfectionistic in their execution, forms that she began painting in the late 1950s and stayed with for a considerable amount of time – or to the softer work of her later years whose perfection is of a less exacting but more sublime nature, one asks *how* our response to her work is shaped by such knowledge. One might ask if the grids – tightly bonded, rigorously executed, and ultimately invariable in their method of execution – are to be viewed as defending against the intrusions of obsessive ideation or hallucinatory perception, against the thinking she worked hard at obliterating, or against the periodic depression from which she suffered: "I have practiced not thinking, until now I can not think for the whole morning," she told an interviewer. "In fact, I do not think when I paint." She kept her mind empty, she said, and chose not to live in the zone of depression that lies "below the line." Instead, she said, "I just live in the upper section with love and beauty and happiness."[28] One is tempted, in short, to ask how much the rigorously executed grids constituted a triumph over internal fragmentation, quiet over excessive stimulation. Might their calm have provided tranquility against the turmoil of hallucinations and other forms of chaos? Or did they rather have something to do with her exceedingly self-effacing tendencies and extreme asceticism? Are the harmonious, blissful even, late paintings – the "imageless images" – related to the trance-like catatonia she experienced? Or, conversely, given their chronology, do they exhibit the lessening of the hold of her illness over her life, an illness that did, as is sometimes the case, increasingly abate over time?

At one point, Martin tried not talking for three years; at other times, she limited her food intake to two or three items for extended periods. Renunciation for Martin was a path to purity, much like her spiritual penchant for Buddhism, much like the ecstatic formlessness of her late art. If she identified with Abstract Expressionism far more than Minimalism, it was that, like her refutation of the material world, she sought to empty her mind of thought. Martin opposed the sin of pride and egoism. Was this but a manifestation of the ennui, the negative symptomology of many with schizophrenia? Was it an expression of the wish to recover the unity of the oceanic (briefly referred to in Chapter Four)? Martin herself wrote, "Abstract or non objective feelings are a very important part of our lives. Personal emotions and sentimentality are anti-art."[29] What I refer to as her "imageless images" seem to suggest a pull toward the earliest phases of life when symbiotic fusion defines experience. (And, as Nancy Olsen has noted, several of the titles of her paintings suggest this as well: *Loving Love, Milk River, Falling Blue, I Love the Whole World, With My Back to the World*, and *Gratitude*, among others.[30]) Moreover, what was most important to Martin in the work of other artists she admired – particularly that of Clyfford Still, Mark Rothko, Jackson Pollock, and Barnett Newman[31] – was the sense of anonymity and the sense of spacelessness she found there. This was what she was after even in the limitless adjacent squares she configured *ad infinitum* to reach the ultimate state of non-configuration. However measured the format, nothing is more silent and silencing, more disciplined and demanding (and thereby restrictive and withholding), than the grids she repeatedly executed.

Once again, the question is this: How do we view these paintings knowing of Martin's schizophrenia? What does our awareness of Martin's psychosis lend, if anything, to our experience of her work? And how might it detract from it? Does it instill within our seeing an appreciation of the extent to which her intense exploration of the grid may have helped her to feel more in control? And, if so, does that matter? Might knowing of a need to distill something affirmative from the catatonic states she experienced constrict how we respond to her painting? Might linking to her illness the philosophy she mightily managed to uphold despite the suffering the illness caused her, a philosophy akin "to a gospel," a philosophy "of happiness,"[32] as one critic put it, strain our responsiveness? How do we view Martin's paintings aware of her engagement with the "oceanic feeling," the egoless union of the infant with the world before it learns there are others in the world as well? Does it deepen our appreciation of her visual art, provoke some other kind of pleasure, or detract from it in some way? Fear, stigma, empathy, and more – all may enter the picture, metaphorically speaking, for better or for worse.

What if we knew, when reading Beckett's poem "What is the Word," the kind of brain damage he had suffered? What if we knew it was the result of a stroke, Parkinson's disease, or some other neurodegenerative illness? What if we knew of the connection between the specific creation of that poem and aphasia? Might that affect or impede upon the pleasure we take from his literary art?

The answers, of course, are as variable as the number of viewers and readers. But the point is this: Cognition and feeling were long considered independent of each other – emotion was linked to the amygdala and cognition to the prefrontal cortex with insufficient recognition of their interrelation, insufficient recognition of the neural mechanisms inherent in emotional processes. Genes, biological signals, neuronal circuits all play into the complexity of feeling whose sources are unattributable to environment alone. When we resituate the relation of cognition and feeling, the relation between mental processes – with consciousness understood as awareness of feeling as Solms has shown – the affective constitution of aesthetic experience becomes clearer.

Ironically, it is segments of an interview with Agnes Martin's psychiatrist in New Mexico, Dr. Donald Fineberg, that illustrate the point:

> Agnes was the person who taught me to appreciate how modern art affects you. She took me to her studio in Taos and she stood me in front of her canvases and she asked me, "What does that make you feel like?" And I said, "Agnes, I've looked at the stripes for a long time and I'm sorry but I'm just confused" and she laughed out loud. On the back of the canvas, the title was "Confusion." And it worked again: She said,

> "What about this one?" It was pinks and yellows. "It just totally makes me very happy," I said. And the title was "Happiness." It happened three times. The third one was a dark-striped purple… "I don't know, Agnes; it just makes me, I don't know…" It was called "Contemplation."
>
> It's all in the feeling. And because of Agnes I came to appreciate that representational art has the same effect only you are distracted by your frontal lobes because there is a picture in front of you.
>
> And there's a reason why there is one bowl of fruit in a still life that makes you happy, like you want to eat it, and another that reminds you – with the shadows and the forms, the whole structure of what is on the surface, a bowl of fruit – that you're going to die one of these days. Agnes is the one who taught me that and I'm very grateful to her. It has enriched my life.
>
> According to Agnes, it all had to do with how you feel when you are in front of the canvas. Some people made a lot of, you know: Is she trying to contain her psychosis because she made these grids and she switched to stripes? No. Maybe on the deepest abstract level of which she doesn't speak, but it really had to do with changing to what she felt expressed the feeling of the work.
>
> She would simply say, "This is how you feel. I have a feeling; this is what I put on the canvas." And she conveyed it. I mean, you stand in front of a major work of Agnes Martin and it never disappears into the wallpaper. It's incredible that way.[33]

While Martin's work might be seen as displaying the absence, not only of engagement with the external world, but of an inner sense of self, I would concur with her biographer who claims, "It would […] be grossly irresponsible to approach Martin's paintings as 'schizophrenic.'"[34] However informed by isolation and solitude, by the selfless state that plagued her, they were ultimately the expression of feeling before the uncertainty, the unknowing, the ambiguity in which she located the aesthetic dimension of being human, and the feeling of selflessness was what she aspired to reveal in her painting. It is this that renders her abstractions remarkably stimulating of new experiential modes of being for the viewer. "You must discover the artwork that you like, and realize the response that you make to it," she said to artists. "You must especially know the response that you make to your own work. It is in this way that you discover your direction and the truth about yourself. If you do not discover your response to your own work, you miss the reward. You must look at the work and know how it makes you feel." To the non-artist, she said as much: "[Y]ou can make discoveries about yourself by knowing your response to work that you like."[35]

Aesthetic experience is always necessarily personally relevant. But the personal relevance is of interest not only for what the mind has to tell us about art, but what art has to tell us about the workings of the mind. It is there, I would venture, that the real value of exploring the interrelation of psychobiography and art resides. One might consider why a particular artist chose particular individuals as friends, what interests or concerns the artist in question shared with that person or another, and what aspects of the artist's personality come to light when one considers an artist's choice of particular forms or images. "A guiding principle in my research," psychoanalyst and art historian Laurie Wilson has said, "is the conviction that an artist's unconscious fantasies are at the heart of his or her major works and constitute the core of the artist's thematic preoccupations. The means I use to track these unconscious fantasies resemble some methods of clinical psychoanalysis, chiefly the observation of anomalies, as well as consistent patterns of thought and feeling in the artist's life, statements, and work."[36] How justifiable, however, one might ask, is putting the artist on the couch, an artist in whose absence one can offer psychoanalytic knowledge only of their own reactive self?

As though in answer to the question as to why we write psychoanalytically about art, Nancy Princenthal has said that we turn to art to understand how others see things. "And in trying to account for any work's particular strength, and its meaning, we naturally consider the context in which it was made, the influences it reflects (and exerts), the politics and place of the communities in which the artist lived. These are not unfamiliar to art history, even to the formalist art criticism that reigned when Martin's work was first shown and celebrated." "It's not a big step from such contextualization to personal history: family, friends, lovers; emotional states; hardships and triumphs," she continues. "And from there to gossip is not a huge step, either. The slope is steeper and more slippery in a culture as focused as ours is on personality and lurid drama." Obviously, she concludes, "it is not impossible to avoid the plunge."[37] Pathologizing the artist, assuming the existence of certain unconscious fantasies, is to take "the plunge," while tolerating *the ambiguity and multiple determination of the feeling states constitutive of the aesthetic experience and, indeed, of the artwork itself*, as abstract painting in particular invites us to do, is to avoid that plunge and be the better for it.

The late British historian and philosopher of science John Forrester claimed that writing about psychoanalysis is "subject to the same laws and processes as the psychoanalytic situation itself."[38] I would say the same is true of writing about art, that writing about art is "subject to the same laws and processes as the psychoanalytic situation itself." Projection, fantasy, defense, ego, repression – all come into play when writing about art in the frame of the artist's psychobiography. Art need not, moreover, emanate from unconscious striving for reparation however encumbered an artist's biography may be by relational trauma. One questions the value of interpretation that seeks not to serve the work of art but usurp its place, as does psycho-historical criticism based on what Susan Sontag, over half a century ago, called "the highly dubious theory that a work of art is composed of items of content." Such interpretation, Sontag so rightly claimed, "violates art" by making it "into an article for use, for arrangement into a mental scheme of categories."[39] Such is the determinism that the post postmodern era in which we now reside must seek to avoid.

Post Postmodernism: Averting Crisis

"Before the problem of the creative artist analysis must, alas, lay down its arms," Freud famously wrote in 1928.[40] The analyst, to put it otherwise, must be humble before the artist whose creative drive was seemingly incomprehensible. The interrelation between art and psychoanalysis does lie beyond the biographical. It lies outside the determinism, the causality, sought by those indulging in psychobiographical explanations of works of art, as Freud himself revealed in "Leonardo Da Vinci and a Memory of His Childhood." Given the intimate connection of talent and sublimation, "we must admit," he wrote in that celebrated essay of 1910, "that the nature of the artistic function is [...] inaccessible to us along psycho-analytic lines." And this: "We must stake out in a quite general way the limits which are set to what psychoanalysis can achieve in the field of biography [...]. The material at the disposal of a psycho-analytic enquiry consists of the data of a person's life-history: on the one hand the chance circumstances of events and background influences, and, on the other hand, the subject's reported reactions." Behavior is explanatory, in other words, by an understanding of the "combined operation of constitution and fate, of internal forces and external powers."[41] The creation of art, however, both content and style, was deemed fundamentally psychoanalytically uninterpretable. "Instincts and their transformations are at the limit of what is discernible by psycho-analysis," he concluded. "From that point it gives place to biological research."[42]

Since Freud's day an ever-increasing number of neuroscientists and neuroaestheticians have revealed much through the biology of affect, which is to say the structural and chemical mechanisms relevant both to the creative impulse psychodynamically viewed as a sublimatory defense and to our reception of the artwork in which it results. An increasing number of neuroscientists and neuroaestheticians have brought to light the biology of perception as well. Yet the question of how our understanding of aesthetic experience is impacted by this substantial increase in the understanding of affect and perception remains insufficiently explored. Why? Psychobiography retains an *uninformed* pull on the critical assessment of art. Why? For lack of recognition that perceptual experience, the sensory encounter, is not intrinsically pleasure-related. For lack of recognition of the contextualization of association. Listen, once again, to Solms: "[T]here is a big difference between the feeling of affects and the associative valancing of externally perceived objects [...]. The difference is this: the affects are inborn but the balancing of external percepts is *acquired*. The visual and other perceptual qualities of percepts become 'associated' with affects in the empiricist sense." For evidence, one need look no further than did Solms in writing of the association of "certain colours with certain feelings," that between "the color red with ripe fruit or hot fires," between, for example, pleasure and danger.[43]

"Oculocentrism," like "corticocentrism," is, as its suffix would imply and as has already been stressed, reductionistic. For inference based upon memory and learning, as upon context, is what transforms our sensory engagement with our environs and not merely the cortex, or at least not merely the way we have long thought the cortex did. Solms, Damasio, Panksepp, and others have taken us far on this neurobiological path. And the implications are vast. Perhaps most significant among them is that of "corrective inference," as Solms refers to our habitual means of perceiving in accordance with expectation: "What you perceive is not the same thing as the input that arrives from your senses. What you perceive is an inference. And the materials from which that inference is derived are for the most part your cortical predictive model derived from the past (i.e., expected) experiences."[44]

How much this tells us about our experience of art! How much this tells us about the motivations of those termed "modernist" and "postmodernist" artists alike, as of the reception of their work! Expectation, perception, correction: All are terms profoundly related to the pleasure, or lack of pleasure, experienced in our viewing, reading, listening to art.

What needs further recognition, however, is that this extension of probability theory, this expansion of Bayes' theorem, is but another way of recognizing what Jacques Garelli described as the inseparability of a color viewed from the order of the color itself, an order which is never stabilized in a definitive identity. It is but another way of recognizing the relation of objective phenomena to subjective experience, the relation of matter (such as the painting or poem) to the affect enjoined with its perception, and the relation of such phenomena to the world. *It is this that necessitates a reevaluation of the modern, a reevaluation of the postmodern, and the notion of creativity itself.* It is the very reason why the philosophers whose names have appeared in this book – Merleau-Ponty, Garelli, Maldiney, and Simondon – turned to painting and poetry, as Solms turned to the example of color, to illustrate the assignment of feeling to one's surrounds, as Panksepp did to illustrate the activation of emotional systems by music. *And it is what defines the era of the post postmodern: a time in which the errors of determinism and the inferences in which they result risk being not recognized for what they are; a time in which the determinism of the cortico-centrist, of the cognitively oriented neuroscientist who fails to recognize the role of feeling in consciousness, in which the determinism of the psychobiographer with the absent artist on the couch, risks remaining insufficiently exposed.* It is what defines the crises of modernism (the struggle to find new values among those rejected), of postmodernism (the struggle to locate the origins of meaning), and the post postmodern (the struggle to restore humanism to an increasingly dehumanizing and uncertain world).

"If form were truly given and predetermined, there would be no genesis, plasticity, or uncertainty relative to the future of a physical system, an organism, or a perceptive field; but this is precisely not the case. There is a genesis of forms just as there is a genesis of life," Simondon asserted.[45] There is a genesis of forms resulting from affective as well as perceptual associations, which is why aesthetic experience is just that: an *experience* of art. That, moreover, is why there is *uncertainty* in artistic form – as in that of the human itself – instability necessitating acceptance both of Beckett's "mess" and "Friston's Law." As Bruno Latour says, "If the human does not possess a stable form, it is not formless for all that." And this:

> The expression "anthropomorphic" considerably underestimates our humanity. We should be talking about morphism. Morphism is the place where technomorphisms, zoomorphisms, phusimorphisms, ideomorphisms, theomomorphisms, sociomorphisms, psychomorphisms, all come together. Their alliances and their exchanges, taken together, are what define the *anthropos*. A weaver of morphisms – isn't that enough of a definition? The closer the *anthropos* comes to this distribution, the more human it is. The farther away it moves, the more it takes on multiple forms in which its humanity quickly becomes indiscernible, even if its figures are those of the person, the individual or the self. By seeking to isolate its form from those it churns together, one does not defend humanism, one loses it.[46]

Referring to his conception of being as a process of individuation, to his theory of potentiality as founded on the interrelation of the individual with their surroundings (technological as well as human), Simondon similarly deflates the anthropocentric view:

> Such a theory doesn't merely seek to explain the genesis of individuated beings and to propose a vision of individuation; it attempts to make of individuation the foundation of an amplifying becoming and therefore places individuation between an initial state of the unresolved being and the entrance into the resolutive path of becoming; individuation is not the result of becoming or something produced in becoming, but becoming in itself insofar as becoming is the being's becoming.[47]

How not to conclude with Solms' comprehensive assessment: "The link between affectivity on the one hand and Helmholtz's 'free energy' on the other seems to identify a red thread through Freud's work, linking him backward to Helmholtz and forward [...] to Friston."[48] But need the understanding of aesthetic experience in terms of what Solms terms "the rediscovery of the embodied, instinctual brain – which must of necessity be constrained by the cognitive brain, with its predictive modeling" lead to the conclusions too readily drawn by those privileging cognition over affect, over the experience that is feeling? "It is difficult to imagine," writes Solms, "how the neuroscience of the future can be anything but psychodynamic."[49] So, too, aesthetics with its conjoined neuroscientific and insufficiently acknowledged ontological foundation that prevents the psychodynamic from being thetically reduced to the objectifying fixity of the psychohistorical. Describing the phenomenon of color as the integration of the seer into the field of the seen – as the occurrence of color in accordance with the qualia of color, with the feeling of perceiving it – Garelli describes exploration of one's most intimate self to reach a similar conclusion.[50]

"What Beckett shares with the post-structuralists," literary theorist Terry Eagleton has written, is "a fear of determinacy." So, too, Asse and others whose art is oriented toward "a creative sort of nothingness," a nothingness that "is the foundation of any authentic ethics or politics." As Eagleton explains, "In the wake of Hitler and the Gulag, there is something profoundly disturbing about the *proposition*. It belongs to a grammar of violence. Too many have perished of absolute truth in the modern age. Certainty can be lethal, but irony and ambiguity can act as antidotes."[51] This is to say that curiosity and creativity can combat the toxicity. At the same time, however, as it has been my purpose to show, certainty is preferable, necessary even, when the antithesis pertains not to conviction but to an understanding of the nature of one's surrounds, of the world, for it is then that crisis of a biological as opposed to ethical or political nature ensues.

As stated at the start of this book, *Where Art Meets Science* was initially to be its subtitle. And where art meets science, it has been my purpose to show, is in philosophy. As Damasio has said, "Philosophical inquiry and science developed from the same homeostatic cloth." Feelings impel the investigations of each: Whether fear before the crises of war, climate change, and more, or pleasure as learning predictively takes place, feeling is what induces curiosity and impels creativity. "The homeostatic benefits of philosophical inquiry and scientific observation are endless," Damasio writes in asserting the obvious but insufficiently recognized.[52] Philosophical inquiry, the humanities more generally, allow us to think about what it is to be human, in what the pleasures – as experienced aesthetically, for instance – and crises of which we are at risk, consist. In neuroscience and psychoanalysis, in neuropsychoanalysis, as in artistic expression whatever the aesthetic arena, it all comes down to feeling. Uncanny is, once again, how I would characterize the convergence in "understanding" that takes place both in science and art rendering philosophy, with its exploration of the subjective uncertainty of the once familiar acknowledged by Freud, the meeting point at hand.

Notes

1 Marjorie Perloff, "Modernism after Postmodernism," presented by the Center for Creative and the Critical, Ashoka University and literaryactivism.com, in partnership with TORCH and the India International Centre, Delhi, 2022.

2 Samuel Beckett, "Dante . . . Bruno . Vico . . Joyce" in *Disjecta*, ed. Ruby Cohn (Grove Press, 1984), 27.
3 Maurice Blanchot, *The Writing of the Disaster*, trans. Ann Smock (University of Nebraska Press, 1986/1995), n.p.
4 Joseph Kuzma, *Internet Encyclopedia of Philosophy*. https://iep.utm.edu/maurice-blanchot/#SH3b
5 Kuzma, *Internet Encyclopedia of Philosophy*.
6 Daniel Albright, "Series Editor's Foreword," in *Samuel Beckett and the Arts*, ed. Lois Oppenheim (Routledge, 1999/2021), viii.
7 Albright, "Series Editor's Foreword," ix.
8 Albright, "Series Editor's Foreword," xii.
9 Jean-Paul Sartre, *Qu'est-ce que la littérature?* (Gallimard, 1948), 15.
10 Alice Jardine, *At the Risk of Thinking* (Bloomsbury, 2020), 245.
11 Cf. Richard Begam, *Samuel Beckett and the End of Modernity* (Stanford University Press, 1996), 14.
12 Antonio Damasio, *The Strange Order of Things*: Life, Feeling, and the Making of Culture (Pantheon, 2018), 179–81.
13 Damasio, *The Strange Order of Things*, 218.
14 Gilbert J. Rose, *Necessary Illusion: Art as Witness* (International Universities Press, Inc., 1996), 107.
15 Jason Baskin, *Modernism beyond the Avant-Garde: Embodying Experience* (Cambridge University Press, 2019), 10.
16 Christopher Rothko, *Mark Rothko: From the Inside Out* (Yale University Press, 2015), 19, 32.
17 Solms, "The Conscious Id," *Neuropsychoanalysis*, 15:1, 5–19, DOI: 10.1080/15294145.2013.10773711.
18 Vittorio Gallese, "Aesthetics and the Unconscious: Toward an Embodied Neuroscience of the Image," JAPA 20, no. 10 (2025). DOI: 10.1177/00030651251394305.
19 Gallese, "Aesthetics and the Unconscious."
20 Gallese, "Aesthetics and the Unconscious."
21 Eissler letter dated September 26, 1983 and Greenacre letter dated June 23, 1983 provided by L. Hoffman.
22 Leon Hoffman, "Picasso and the Painter Model Theme: Multiple Identifications and Creative Transformations of Aggressive Conflicts," *International Review of Psycho-Analysis* 11 (1984), 291–300.
23 Gaston Bachelard, *The Poetics of Space*, Foreword to the 1994 edition, trans. Maria Jolas (Beacon Press, 1958/1994), xvii–xviii (emphasis added).
24 Michael Coffey, *Beckett's Children: A Literary Memoir* (Evergreen Review Books, 2024), 35.
25 Coffey, *Beckett's Children: A Literary Memoir*, 37, 33.
26 Sander Van de Cruys, Jacopo Frascaroli, and Karl Friston, "Order and Change in Art: Towards an Active Inference Account of Aesthetic Experience," *Philosophical Transactions of the Royal Society* (2023). B 379:20220411. doi:10.1098/rstb.2022.0411
27 Yayoi Kusama, *Infinity Net: The Autobiography of Yayoi Kusama*, trans. Ralph McCarthy, Smithsonian Libraries. https://siris libraries.si.edu/ipac20/ipac.jsp?&profile=liball&source=~!silibraries&uri=full=3100001~!1108965~!0#focus
28 Video with interview, camera, and editing Mary Lance. Shown in conjunction with the Agnes Martin retrospective exhibit at the Guggenheim Museum, New York, October 7, 2016–January 11, 2017.
29 Agnes Martin, "Beauty is the Mystery of Life," https://www.artbook.com/blog-excerpt-agnes-martin-beauty-is-the-mystery-of-life.html#:~:text=Ask%20yourself:%20%E2%80%9CWhat%20kind%20of,and%20sentimentality%20are%20anti%2Dart

30 Nancy Olsen, meeting of Western New England Psychoanalytic Society, April 28, 2018.
31 See Nancy Princenthal, *Agnes Martin: Her Life and Art* (Thames & Hudson, 2015), 210.
32 Peter Schjeldahl, "Drawing Lines," *The New Yorker* (October 17, 2016): 107, 106.
33 Personal interview with Donald Fineberg, Jan. 9, 2020, unpublished.
34 Princenthal, *Agnes Martin: Her Life and Art*, 173.
35 Martin, "Beauty is the Mystery of Life."
36 Laurie Wilson, "Alberto Giacometti's *Woman with Her Throat Cut*: Multiple Meanings and Methodology," *The Annual of Psychoanalysis* 26 (1999): 148.
37 Nancy Princenthal, "With Her Back to the World and Her Face to the Camera," *Brooklyn Rail*, November 2013, https://brooklynrail.org/2013/11/criticspage/with-her-back-to-the-world-and-her-face-to-the-camera/.
38 John Forrester, *Thinking in Cases* (Polity Press 66, 2017). Qtd. by Paul Shimmel in his review of the book, *JAPA* 65, no. 6 (2017): 1138.
39 Susan Sontag, *Against Interpretation* (Farrar, Straus and Giroux, 1961), 10, 12.
40 Sigmund Freud, "Dostoevsky and Parricide," *Standard Edition*, vol. 21, 177.
41 Sigmund Freud, "Leonardo Da Vinci and a Memory of His Childhood," *Standard Edition*, vol. 11, 136, 134–5, 135.
42 Freud, "Leonardo Da Vinci and a Memory of His Childhood," 136.
43 Mark Solms, *The Hidden Spring: A Journey to the Source of Consciousness* (W.W. Norton, 2021), 235.
44 Solms, *The Hidden Spring: A Journey to the Source of Consciousness*, 219.
45 Gilbert Simondon, *Individuation in Light of Notions of Form and Information*, trans. Taylor Adkins (University of Minnesota Press, 2020), 258.
46 Bruno Latour, *We Have Never Been Modern*, trans. Catherine Porter (Harvard University Press, 1993), 137.
47 Simondon, *Individuation in Light of Notions of Form and Information*, 367.
48 Mark Solms, "The Conscious Id," *Neuropsychoanalysis* 15, no. 1 (2013): 18. DOI:10.1080/15294145.2013.10773711
49 Solms, "The Conscious Id," 18.
50 See Jacques Garelli, "Voir ceci et voir selon," in *Merleau-Ponty, Phénoménologie et expériences*, ed. Marc Richir and Étienne Tassin (Jérôme Million, 1992) (trans. mine).
51 Terry Eagleton, "Foreword: Nothing," in *New, Beckett and Nothing: Trying to Understand Beckett*, ed. Daniela Caselli (Manchester University Press, 2010), xxv.
52 Damasio, *The Strange Order of Things*, 182–83.

Conclusion : The Devalorization of the Intellectual in the Twenty-First Century

"**Science** ***n.*** [OF., fr. L. *scientia*, fr. *sciens, -entis*, pres. part. of *scire* to know [...].] A branch of study which is concerned with observation and classification of facts, especially with the establishment (and, strictly, the quantitative formulation) of verifiable general laws, chiefly by induction and hypotheses; as, the biological, historical, and mathematical *sciences*."[1]

Interestingly, at Oxford University the sciences formerly referred to "a group of studies mainly in the works of ancient and modern philosophers."[2] Today, however, in line with the definition above, they are everywhere distinguished from all branches of learning "regarded as primarily conducive to culture"[3]; in other words, the humanities. Are the natural sciences and humanities forever to remain at the antipodes of one another? Or might we already be at the threshold of a (re)unification (think of the Renaissance) in the investigation of the role played by the brain in the emergence of mind, in the valorization of consciousness as dependent upon feeling, as fundamentally affective? Might we, in fact, already be in the trenches of interdisciplinarity in the exploration of *why* we are driven to know and to create (to SEEK, to PLAY), in the exploration of *how* we view the painting and read the poem? Neuronal networks as related to affect as well as memory and awareness, neurotransmitters as related to these circuits and to the contextualizing experience that (literally) drives them: Attention to such interplay, that between anatomy and chemistry, has never been more necessary as uncertainty continues to unsettle us, psychodynamically as well as homeostatically speaking, and crisis destabilizes our sense of who we are. Attention to such interplay has never been more intriguing as we perceive the transition in process from metapsychology to "meta*neuro*psychology," from psychoanalysis to neuropsychoanalysis, as from aesthetics to neuroaesthetics and "neuropsychoaesthetics," and move, epistemologically speaking, beyond the dualizing tendencies of our past.

As Solms has written, "There can be few better examples of the limits that the hard-won knowledge of the Humanities places on cognitive neuroscience than the radically subjective nature of the mind. This makes it impossible to have a physical science of psychology." Indeed, "'scientific psychology' is only

DOI: 10.4324/9781003566755-7

an oxymoron if 'scientific' is considered synonymous with 'physical.'" As he further explains, "we cannot have a scientific psychology if we limit ourselves to spatial concepts [...] and if we disregard the peremptory power of affect, because we thereby disregard the motivational forces that so easily distort the supposed neutrality of 'objective' spatial cognition." Psychoanalysis, defined as "a science of the mind that does not consider 'scientific' to be synonymous with 'physical,'" relies "heavily on empathy as a method of investigation." And it does so because it maintains "proper respect for feelings."[4]

It is the "proper respect for feelings" that leads one to conclude as to the reality of aesthetic objects – objects "actually as dead as doornails" – and the futility of analyzing from either a physicalist or psychohistorical perspective what is devoid of a psyche. Of course, there is much to be said, it almost goes without saying, for consideration of the artist's life experience. But such consideration must not diminish the potential for evolution, for emergence and transformation, which is to say that it must not reductively ignore the interrelation of the affective with the ontological, that which constitutes the phenomenological *reality* of the "imaginary" work of art.

Inquiring as to why some need to find in the abstract the figurative, moreover, as Christopher Rothko has done, not only takes us beyond the psychobiographical reductivism of that critical perspective, but brings us closer to that very "reality." "Is there something inherently unstable in abstraction? Something threatening? Something ominous?" he has asked.[5] Why do some need "to make the painted image *something,* to read it as a reference to a thing we can recognize," a need that "takes us away from both the experience of the painting itself and our experience of ourselves in the context of that painting," he has wondered.[6] In agreement with him, I would add: Is it not far more interesting to ask what abstract paintings, such as those by Mark Rothko and others, can tell us of the viewer rather than the artist, what the "imageless image" of Agnes Martin and others may tell us about ourselves? "Rothko paintings raise [...] existential fears because their simplicity, their vast open planes, can suggest the void," Rothko's son continues. "If you look squarely into the Rothko void, however, its fullness becomes much more evident. There is nothing nihilistic about these paintings, not even the most austere late works." But here is the point: "To communicate with a Rothko painting is to *feel* that something, to experience the substance of being, the substance of our humanness."[7]

And there is this: Just as the viewer's or reader's psychically dynamic and sensory-neural response to, arousal from and interaction with, a visual or literary artwork at any given moment is highly significant, such is the artist's own perpetual becoming by way of imagination, by way of creativity understood as the reduction of uncertainty through embodiment in the image, in the movement we see and the beats we hear. Implanted in the work, they capture perception and action in feeling. Indeed, we have seen just how reductive and deterministic psychobiography can be and how error-ridden as well insofar as what is removed from the psychohistorical is precisely the very temporality that makes the "physics of sentience" what it is, what makes the biology of the MindBrain what it is. What is removed is the functional dimension that led Freud to detect what Solms terms "the ontological substrate of language" and to conclude that it is "'virtual.'" Comparable in its functionality to hysteria, Freud's earliest focus which he found to exist "not within the elements of the nervous system but between them," the ontology of language is operative.[8] So, too, the work of art whatever the genre, as perhaps most evident in the abstractions of modern art from Abstract Expressionism to the Theater of the Absurd.

Just as the "scientific 'object' discovered at the end of research" is inseparable "from the path of the thought and the operative processes that have led to revealing and constructing it,"[9] as Garelli put it, aesthetic experience is inextricably linked to its formation, the temporalizing process of ontogenesis, which is to say that its creation is indivisible from its dynamic co-creation as well. That the work of art is irreducible to an object is owed to its irreducibility to a subject as independent of what Garelli terms the "principle of individuation," the "Becoming of mind" that never definitively becomes what it is. Not becoming what it is, however, is but another oxymoron, for it never becomes other than what it is: that which evolves *in time*, "a process intrinsic to the formations of individuals, who are never completed, never fixed, never stable, but always accomplishing in their evolution an individuation that structures them," to further cite Garelli on Simondon.[10] Therein lies the meaning of what we would do well to term "neuropsychoaesthetics," the value of what we would do well to recognize as the *experiencing* of art.

*

More than a century ago, John Dewey wrote that "the most notable distinction between living and inanimate things is that the former maintain themselves by renewal." This "principle of continuity through renewal," as Dewey called it, referenced, of course, human biology, the homeostatic imperative underlying the behavioral responsiveness of every individual. "With the renewal of physical existence," Dewey explained, "goes [...] the re-creation of beliefs, ideals, hopes, happiness, misery, and practices"; in other words, the affective and related consequences afforded by the processing of prediction and the minimization of uncertainty as concordant with physical well-being.[11]

It has been the purpose of this book to explore *how biology*, as the primary determinant of behavior (determinant as used here not to be confused with the non-biological social determinisms of convention, economics, the psychobiographical, and other reductionisms), *relates to aesthetic experience*. It has been my objective to explore what remains when "the workings of thought" are accepted as irreducible to "the workings of the neurones" (as François Noudelmann put it and I cited at the start), when creativity and imagination are accepted as irreducible to visual circuitry or to the subliminal recognition that is the crux of embodied simulation, reducible neither to the ocular nor to the motoric, however much each system may be activated in the resonance at play in the experiencing of art. Rather, it is how the workings of such neural processes, *when regarded* as *essential to affect as the foundation of consciousness, when regarded as essential to the intentionality of perception, to the directedness of drive,* are constitutive of aesthetic experience, that it has been my intent to consider.

"In psychoanalysis," Henry Markman has written, "in the encounter with new feeling new qualities of being emerge – in oneself and within the dyad." Citing the painting of Robert Motherwell, he defines an ontological comparability between psychoanalysis and aesthetic experience: "The brush strokes are alive with becoming."[12] What defines the *becoming* of any experiential phenomenon, be it maturational, aesthetic, psychoanalytic, or other, is the dynamic process of individuation, as my focus on Garelli, Maldiney, and Simondon was meant to show. And what constitutes this fundamentally ontogenetic perspective are the tensions, the sensorial rhythms, the energy or drive that renders the encounter with art necessarily intersubjective and this despite the absent subject, that of the artist not dissimilar from that of the analyst (most conspicuously so in a truly Freudian analytic frame). "What is the word?" asked Samuel Beckett. What is the word when one has difficulty finding the word, perhaps because of aphasia? What is the word when the word and its associations are repressed? What is the word, the right word, that will succeed in stimulating aesthetic pleasure? What is the word that, when used in a literary way, is comparable to the brush stroke, to the musical note, and as materially irreducible as they are? What is the word used creatively to constitute a work of art that is in itself lifeless, subjectless, "actually as dead as doornails"? This is the question posed by modern art, and "modern thought generally" as Merleau-Ponty demonstrated, that "obliges us to admit a truth which does not resemble things, which is without any external model and without any predestined instruments of expression, and which is nevertheless truth."[13]

I began the first chapter with the notion that the implicit if not explicit investigation of *sentio ergo sum* (as opposed to the dichotomizing Cartesian *cogito ergo sum*) would appear preliminary to any consideration of the making and viewing, reading, or listening to art. What I hope to have demonstrated is how drive theory (as articulated by Freud and re-visioned by Solms and others) coupled with the Free Energy Principle (more specifically, with predictive coding minus several erroneously drawn conclusions) contributes to our understanding of aesthetic experience. In as much as a painting cannot be reduced to the space it occupies any more than a poem can be reduced to the words appearing on the page or a symphony to a musical score, it is through the very act of perceiving, through the awareness that is consciousness and the feeling implicated therein, that the being of the artwork unfolds. But perception alone does not account for the experiencing of a work of art. Hegel described the process by which the object is negated in its limited individuality, preserved in its essential being, and elevated to a higher reality. Thus is the ontology of the work of art revealed. Mallarmé's famous statement "Je dis: une fleur! [...] l'absente de tous bouquets" may be said to illustrate this, the Hegelian *Aufhebung*. So, too, Heidegger located this *becoming* of aesthetic creation beyond the duality of representation, situating "I think" in Dasein, in the *being there* of "I am," which in turn situated the processes at work in art in the viewer/reader/listener's own ego projection in space and time. *In this integration unfolds the wonder, the curiosity, and thereby crisis-evading and creative encounter that constitutes the very relation that is the experience of art.*

I continued in the chapters that followed with the notion that crisis, from Husserl to Sartre, Kristeva, and others, emanates from inattention to subjectivity and the determinism to which that omission gives rise. So, too, neuroscientists have bemoaned the critical omission of subjectivity from the study of the brain, an omission that means, according to Panksepp and Biven, that "we cannot simply approach the study of brain functions with traditional third-person tools of science." As they explain: "The mind is not a neutral thing like a stone in a field. It has a point of view, an I-ness. And every viewpoint that really matters is strongly tinged with affect. To see the Brain-Mind for what it really is, we must deal with subjectivity ever more effectively in neuroscientific terms. When we do an accurate archeology of the mind, we find affective experience at the mind's foundation." Indeed, as they further observe, "Affect is the very heart of what the brain does when it processes external 'rewards' and 'punishments.'"[14] Neubauer, Abrams, and Balzert's unpublished study similarly reveals that it is such affective processing of life experience that allows for development, for the "pull forward" that constitutes maturation. And, as Solms convincingly demonstrates with regard to the mind-brain relation, affect is what consciousness itself (not congruent with the intellect as is traditionally and erroneously misconstrued) is all about.[15]

So it is, as it has been my objective to show, that the source of creativity lies in its neurobiological function, which is to say its goal-oriented, motivational predisposition toward the satisfaction of curiosity. As I have stated in Chapter 3 and elsewhere,[16] whatever the verbal or visual image produced, however many times the image destroyed and remade, rather than as a re-presentation of an external reality, the neurophilosophical perspective, like the metaneuropsychological, allows for its understanding as a response to endogenous demands. As I also stressed earlier, that the work of art is a manifestation of unconscious need, fantasy, and wish is not in any way invalidated by recognition of this understanding. If, as Freud wrote, "past, present and future are strung together [...] on the thread of the wish that runs through them," what Solms offers in his updating of Freud – in his "Revision of Drive Theory," in his "New Project for a Scientific Psychology," in *The Hidden Spring: A Journey to the Source of Consciousness*, to name but three of his many writings – is an understanding of *why*. And now we ask: What is the "meta*neuro*psychological" *raison d'être* of that novel or poem, of that painting? It is *purpose: the* *endogenous, fundamentally affective, and self-organizing objective of self-preservation achieved through the prediction of outcome.* It is the Deweyesque "principle of continuity through renewal" accounted for in the pleasure of fulfillment afforded by the aesthetic experience.

If there is a primary take away from this exploration it is that the dialectic of the imaginative and the real are no more oppositional than the body and the mind. We know from epigenetics that life experience can alter the expression of some genes leaving the DNA intact, as the observational twins study with which I began reveals and the neuropsychoanalytic view of the MindBrain confirms. Similarly, how we understand imagination, how we understand aesthetic experience – even when form presides over image for the aesthetic "object"'s being so abstract as to be unrelatable to anything outside it – requires that we no longer ignore the temporal dimension of aesthetic experience. How we understand aesthetic experience requires that the relation of one's affective interaction, one's affective integration, with a work of art exceed the temporality of a given moment in time in favor of the temporalization of the artwork itself. This is to say that the energizing, the neuronal arousal constituting the apperception of the artwork, the relational dimension and intentionalizing force, is the very drive at play in the work's being in-formation, its temporalizing feature indissociable from its ontology.

What I have aimed to demonstrate, in part, is why the relation between neuropsychoanalysis and other disciplines is proving increasingly significant. Cognitive and affective neuroscience, psychoanalysis, and philosophy are all deeply related to the literary and visual arts, both experientially and theoretically. And the psychosocial, political, cultural, economic, anthropological, art historical, and other determinants are in some measure inherent in the creative use of the mind, from fantasy to aesthetic expression. Yet, however affixed to the real, the subjective transcends the deterministic by virtue of the very forces that drive imagination: joy and curiosity, which imply PLAY and SEEKING, the forces that take one beyond pleasure to the satiation of need. Garelli, as a philosopher writing about art and a poet as well, went so far as to claim that poetic activity, like all art, is self-revelatory: it unveils itself in the act of its unveiling, its opening onto the world. And however paradoxical – "the poetic work renders present that which opens a presence"[17] – this unveiling emits a kind of nostalgia, a reminiscence put in high relief by the neuroscientist's theoretical understanding, whatever the perspective, of the experience of abstract art. Abstracted from a totality in itself un-representable, abstract painting exemplifies the experiencing of all art in its unavoidable omission of a kind coherence to be but unconsciously, if nostalgically, recalled. Whether in the delineation of such experience through the emphasis, à la Zeki, on the ocular or in its repeated contextualization, by Gallese, as "social practice," there is what Christopher Rothko comparably recognized as a "nostalgia for unity." At once individual and universal (to the extent that subjectivity can be presumed to reside in the other), it is this that led John Day, Agnes

Martin, Geneviève Asse, and Mark Rothko, like Samuel Beckett, John Cage, and so many others, to seek expansion in the minimal, harmony in the discordant.

As I noted in the Preface, Christopher Rothko wrote that his father's "search for unity, and the society's as well, may be an attempt to fend off an incipient existential crisis – to find constancy and meaning in the face of increasing entropy,"[18] anticipating (unknowingly) the value of applying to aesthetic experience Friston's notion of predictive processing. Such is the "nostalgia for unity," such is the nostalgia of which Garelli, in the phenomenological lineage of Merleau-Ponty and others, wrote when considering the ontology of the movement from absence to presence, from silence to expression, that is the achievement of the creative imagination. In the delineation of the spatiotemporal unity that this "nostalgia" implies, the ambiguity in which all artistic expression resides (as evidenced in this very notion) was also put in high relief by Abstract Expressionism and other modern art. And to the extent that such an aesthetic was initially rejected, one may conclude as to the incipient rejection of the non-deterministic, non-dichotomizing paradigmatic cultural shift presenting itself at the time. To the extent that the insufficiency of the Cartesian subject-object dichotomy is overcome by the remembrance of lived experience and the learning it brings within it, overcome by that to which Friston's notion of predictive coding subscribes, we are obliged to recall with Solms what "Most cognitive scientists working within the predictive processing paradigm forget – all too readily": namely, "that the mind is *embodied*."[19] If not functionally/organically so, the sensory and affective are also embodied in the expression to which such experience (perceptual and emotional) gives form. So, too, are the sensory and affective embodied in the spatiotemporal dynamic of the image (or the "imageless image" of abstraction), in the sound of music or the movement of the dancer. *And this is where neuroaesthetics and psychoanalysis, like brain and mind, reveal their very connection.* Devoid of a subject, the work of art is nonetheless *experienced* and it is in that subjective experience, in the memory and learning embedded in its creation and reception, that the neural and mental are conjoined.

The overriding by theoretical and cultural determinisms of the subjective dynamic – of the existential constituent inherent in the experiential phenomenon of aesthetics, in the ontological intertwining of subject and object (the chiasmus Merleau-Ponty so deftly delineated) – led me to disagree with the conclusions of those who, despite other indisputably valuable contributions to neuroaesthetics, maintain that the pleasure of the aesthetic derives from recognition. It is that which led me to reject the conclusions of those who consider that because a "meaningful encounter with visual art starts with visual sensations" and because of "the evolutionary constraints on our visual system," to experience art more deeply, to attain greater satisfaction from it, "inevitably entails a process of recognition and identification."[20] I have also disagreed with those who maintain that the emotional salience of aesthetic experience is limited to the initial encounter with a work of art. Rather, I have agreed with those who, like Simondon, stress that becoming is a dimension of being, one which, as we know from the predictive perspective outlined by Friston and others, is at risk of crisis if the incompatibility of expectancy and surprisal is not resolved. Once again, as the philosopher wrote, "In a theory of the phases of being, becoming is something other than an alteration or a succession of states comparable to a serial development. Becoming is in effect a perpetuated and renovated resolution, an incorporating resolution, proceeding through crises, such that its sense is in its center, not at its origin or its end."[21] Such a theory does not seek merely to explain the genesis of individuation, but the continual and amplifying process that places it between an initial unresolved and thereby threatened state of being and entry into a path of resolution. Focused neither on a result of becoming nor on something produced in becoming, but on *becoming itself as the principle dimension of being*, it allows for "understanding" (per Bohr's reply to Heisenberg) of the integration of feeling (once again, the source of conscious awareness) with the biology of the cellular system that is ours. It allows for "understanding" of the interdisciplinarity of neuroaesthetics and psychoanalysis (or, more precisely, neuropsychoanalysis) with philosophy (or, more precisely, phenomenology) at the core.

It has been my purpose to explore where art meets science and to do so by delineating the interrelation between curiosity and creativity and their integration within neuroaesthetics and psychoanalysis. It has been my objective to explore if such a meeting, seemingly at the expense of something more objectively or positivistically significant, would be so when understood in the existential framework of crisis. Where does this leave one? Perhaps with the realization that pleasure in discovery when understood as the phenomenon it truly is – i.e., a feeling, which is to say a subjective emotional state arising from the relinquishment of the cognitive prerequisite of re-presentation – is life affirming. Perhaps with the realization that pleasure in discovery, aesthetic pleasure, relates not to empathy in as much as the artwork is without feeling, but to *freedom* in the most fundamental – i.e., Sartrean, which is to say humanistic – sense of the word. It was the dawning of modernism that overtly delegitimized determinism and allowed for the articulation, in whatever the genre, of this most fundamental of realities.

*

"The European 'world,'" as Husserl said – or, the Western world, as might be said at present with more currency – "was born from ideas of reason, i.e., from the spirit of philosophy."[22] And the "great danger" with which the world in its entirety was increasingly confronted in the 1930s was said by Husserl to be "weariness." "Weariness" is no doubt part of the increasingly complex devalorization of the intellectual in the twenty-first century, the degradation of the humanities and the disregard for thinking as (in and of itself) that which once inspired respect for learning (in and for itself) before "the spirit of philosophy" was lost. Yet we are faced at this time with the spread of ultra-conservative politics, the raging of war, climate instability, and the rapid surge of artificial intelligence or the posthuman: Each provokes uncertainty, fear even, the feeling that "crisis" is upon us. Why each is occurring, the extent of its reach, should be stimulating much questioning about the barbarism of our species, stimulating curiosity about the socio-political, ecological, and other destabilizing forces. The lack of great numbers of public intellectuals questioning the cultural manifestations of our increasingly non-thought-oriented society itself is worthy of serious reflection.

Already in 1980, *Le Débat*, a leading French journal of the time, published an issue devoted to the question, "Of what will the future intellectual be made?" Introducing the issue, the editors asked, "Of what will one be speaking in the next few years?" "To say what? To whom? In what form?" Addressing the generation of thirty-year-old protesters who had participated in the May 1968 student uprisings, they continued, "You who began demonstrating, how do you see your intellectual activity developing?" Among the essays of contributing writers, one reads of the malaise of the intellectual, of the hate and negation of life deemed never as strong as in the French intelligentsia of the time. And two hopes for the future are formulated by the increasingly controversial co-authors Pascal Bruckner and Alain Finkielkraut as a result: That intellectuals choose truth over immediate notoriety and exhibit a modicum of pragmatism, on the one hand, and that, on the other, the world of books is made to have greater influence on life.[23] With a different objective in mind, Évelyne Grossman wrote almost three decades later of what she called "the anguish of thought." Attributing this "price to be paid [...] for the spark of an idea," for "inspiration," she wrote of "the cruel *experience* of thinking," of the "dizzying prospect of 'how to begin'" so evident in Beckett, so apparent "at the heart of modern writing" overall.[24] But here's the point: *There is a convergence between thinking and creating, between thinking and painting or the making or experiencing of any other form of art. And this convergence, which resides in the minimization of uncertainty, the giving of form to chaos, gets lost in the mind/brain and affective/cognitive dichotomies that some – in this era of the post postmodern, in the interdisciplinary domains of neuroscience and psychoanalysis, neuroscience and aesthetics – are succeeding to obliterate.* Losing sight of this convergence, of this giving of form, however exacting, leaves us before the very risk of crisis against which creative thinking itself, like the expression of aesthetic vision, serves as protection.

We are faced today with the crisis of which Husserl wrote in the lack of compassion between those of our species for whom it is difficult "to feel they can share their growing dread, grief and fear" and, as a result, feel little other than a "harrowing loneliness," to cite psychoanalyst Josephine Wright. We are faced with this crisis as victims of the extraordinary increase in global warming and related ecological realities, victims of those governments "that do not acknowledge or act on the crises."[25] Husserl wrote in *The Crisis* of "communalization," of the meaning of "living-with-one-another," of "co-subjects" and "co-humanity."[26] We are faced at this time with multiple crises deeply related to the lack of awareness of this meaning and the lack of interest in questioning. According to Husserl, there is but a single solution: "transcendental phenomenology with its secure and grounded clarification of the concept of *subjectivity*," as Moran puts it.[27] Indeed, "clarification of the concept of *subjectivity*," as the primary framework of the humanities, is what defines the very juncture of science and art.

It is in the phenomenological tradition of those who, like Merleau-Ponty, Garelli, Simondon, Maldiney, and others, subscribe to *intentionality* as the foundational element of experience, to the perceptual validation of the existential as opposed to the reductionistic and deterministic theorizing of idealism, that art and science are conjoined. It is in the uncovering of the neuroanatomy and chemistry of emotion and in the recognition of the dynamic, experiential, existential dimension of consciousness to which they give rise that the integration of art and science is to be found. The crisis constituted by the breakdown of our culture at large – with the devalorization of thinking, of the humanities, of the humane even – has its origin, according to Husserl, in the "exteriorization" of rationalism, its incorporation or assimilation into "objectivism," by which is meant a disregard for the essence of our culture in community, in the intimacy of beings for each other.[28]

Freud, moreover, was profoundly influenced by Darwin and considered the origin of what he termed "*primal phantasies*" "a phylogenetic endowment."[29] Psychoanalysis is grounded, in fact, in the inheritance of such fantasies, in the notion of the intergenerational transmission of mental states, and Freud considered "the assumption of a collective mind" essential to its development.[30] Clearly we need now, once again, to think in collective terms. Recognition of the intersection of neuroscience and the humanities, of psychoanalysis and the aesthetic – more specifically, neuropsychoanalysis and the neuroaesthetic – leads us from the increasingly barbaric dehumanization of determinism to the humane. And yet, as journalist Maureen Dowd writing in *The New York Times* has noted, however strange it may be, the humanities are weakening just at the moment we most need them. And it is not only the humanities that are becoming of the past, she so rightly claims, but humanity itself. Moreover, artificial intelligence can hardly be our focus, says Dowd, unless we support and grow the intelligence that is not artificial and already in our possession.[31]

The crisis of which Husserl wrote would end only in a complete and utter alienation from the rational "sense of life" (which he equated with "a barbarian hatred of spirit"), alienation from "a heroism of reason," and in a regeneration of the transcendental, of the intentional (in the phenomenological sense of the term).[32] We are faced today with crisis in the renewal of fascist ideology and the undoing of democracy in parts of Europe and the United States. Yet crisis is crisis whether owing to a turning point in the life of an individual or that of a community, a nation, or the world at large. Defenses may certainly be adaptive in temporarily easing fear or other powerfully uncomfortable feelings. Or they may be maladaptive in provoking other emotional difficulties rather than serving to protect. Then again, they may be both. Imagining the worst, while increasing fear and being clearly, as a result, maladaptive, may also serve as a shield against crisis. It may help one who feels helpless (and thereby in crisis) to feel as though they have some measure of control: If I imagine the worst, I will somehow be protected from its really happening as I will have experience of it in advance. The key word here, of course, is "imagine." Imagining otherwise, engaging creatively not with fantasy but with art, serves to thwart negative feelings as well. As Freud famously believed, sublimation was an ego-mature means of deflecting socially unacceptable impulses into morally or otherwise acceptable activity. Others, Jung and Lacan most notably, offered very different ideas of sublimation but the point is that, whatever the perspective, the objective is transformation, whether of unconscious impulses or something else, for the sake of protection, protection against the feelings from which we suffer. And wherever *crisis* (personal and universal, physiological and psychological) takes us, to avoid homeostatic insufficiency we remain *curious* and thereby, to a greater or lesser extent, *creative* unless an alteration in affect disrupts that motivation and jeopardizes our equilibrium. As the interrelations between the physiology of brain and the foundationally affective nature of mind become ever clearer, it is increasingly evident that, in the connectedness of curiosity, creativity, and crisis, art and science converge.

Why, in the midst of war, might music, visual art, or the literary work be needed? Some years ago, the journalist/critic Jason Farago posed a similar question (hardly a new one, but nevertheless...).[33] And, many years prior to his doing so, the critic Margo Jefferson had responded to it in a way that deeply impressed Farago: Art is needed in times of war because imagination is vital to history, she explained. Imagination allows us to determine how the past and future resemble each other; it provides us with the means to ascertain their differences from and/or resemblances to the present.[34] Irreducible to words on the page or the painted canvas, imagination is critical to the vibrancy of the historical record.

In seeking where art and science meet, I have spoken of psychoanalysis or, more accurately, neuropsychoanalysis through a consideration of aesthetic experience. Why? Aesthetic experience, abstract aesthetic experience above all other, with its minimization of the dichotomy between the heuristic and the ontological, engages with the very process constituting neuropsychoanalysis. And it is this that summarizes what I have aimed to explore in this book. Psychoanalytic inquiry cannot be removed from the aesthetic arena. But how causal it is to be viewed is what is in question, not only because the artist is not on the couch, but because the aesthetic image (however "imageless" it may be) is not reducible to what the philosopher Gaston Bachelard called "an echo of the past."[35] The past may resound in an image and, in so doing, stimulate exploration, but in the actuality of its expression, as in the transference, the imaginative dimension so integral to the analytic process, it has its own dynamic ontology.

The dichotomous approach that separates psyche from soma – which is precisely what is eliminated in the neuropsychoanalytic updating of classical Freudian theory – is illustrative of the very determinism, the linear causality, that, as I have aimed to show, defines one highly significant crisis with which we are currently confronted: the dearth not of artistic output, which will forever be part of the human species, but of the valuation of thinking whatever the arena. The devaluation of the intellectual implies a disrespect of the humanities which explore the cultural output of humans and, ultimately a disrespect of the humanitarian, of the humane. Eric Kandel believes, as a reviewer of *The Disordered Mind: What Unusual Brains Tell Us about Ourselves* has observed, that a new kind of humanism – one in which science, from the biology of the mind to the focus on the natural world, intersects with the humanities in their exploration of human experience – is possible.[36] I would supplement that belief with the notion that neuroscience, when emphasizing the affective over the cognitive perspective, offers a connection between science and the humanities such as it is to be found in aesthetic experience, as it has been my purpose to show. Recognition of the fundamental synthesis of neuroaesthetics and psychoanalysis, or more specifically neuropsychoanalysis, is one step toward the revalorization of the thinking mind. Indeed, recognition of the juncture where neuropsychoanalysis and neuroaesthetics come together, recognition of the value of one for the other, takes us one step away from the finitude, the reductionism of a physicalist thinking that is exclusive of the subjective, the affective, and the ontological as well. Our biology, in and of itself, requires such recognition, for, to cite psychoanalyst François Ansermet, "We are biologically determined not to be biologically determined."[37]

Notes

1 Webster's New International Dictionary, 2nd edn (G. & C. Merriam Company, 1956).
2 Webster's New International Dictionary.
3 Webster's New International Dictionary.
4 Mark Solms, "Empathy as Developmental Achievement: Beyond Embodied Simulation," in *Neuroscience and Critique*, ed. Jan De Vos and Ed Pluth (Routledge, 2016), 218.
5 Christopher Rothko, "Ceci n'est pas un frigo," *Mark Rothko: From the Inside Out* (Yale University Press, 2015), 40.
6 Rothko, "Ceci n'est pas un frigo," 45.
7 Rothko, "Ceci n'est pas un frigo," 51.
8 Mark Solms, "'Function' in Functional Neurological Disorders: The Common Ground of Neuroscience and Psychoanalysis," Neuropsychoanalysis 27, no. 1 (2025): 5–18.
9 Jacques Garelli, "Foreword: Introduction to the Problematic of Gilbert Simondon," in Gilbert Simondon, *Individuation in Light of Notions of Form and Information*, trans. Taylor Adkins (University of Minnesota Press, 2020), xvi.
10 Garelli, "Introduction to the Problematic of Gilbert Simondon," xxiv.
11 John Dewey, *Democracy and Education* (The Free Press, 1916), 1–2.

12 Henry Markman, "So Much Depends Upon a Red Stripe," *Psychoanalytic Inquiry* 44, no. 4 (2024): 398–409.
13 Merleau-Ponty, "Indirect Language and the Voices of Silence," 94.
14 Jaak Panksepp and Lucy Biven, The Archeology of Mind: Neuroevolutionary Origins of Human Emotions (W.W. Norton, 2012), 422–23.
15 See Mark Solms, *The Hidden Spring: A Journey to the Source of Consciousness* (W.W. Norton, 2021), chap. 12.
16 Lois Oppenheim, "Commentary on Mark Solms' 'New Project for a Scientific Psychology,'" *Neuropsychoanalysis* 22, no. 1–2 (2021): 87–89.
17 Jacques Garelli, *La gravitation poétique* (Mercure de France, 1966), 9.
18 Christopher Rothko, "Introduction," in Mark Rothko, *The Artist's Reality* (Yale University Press, 2004), xxi.
19 Solms, "'Function' in Functional Neurological Disorders."
20 Ladislav Kesner, "'A Hole in a Piece of Cardboard and Predictive Brain: The Incomprehension of Modern Art in the Light of the Predictive Coding Paradigm," Philosophical Transactions of the Royal Society, 2024, 3. B 379: 20220417. https://doi.org/10.1098/rstb.2022.0417
21 Gilbert Simondon, *L'Individuation psychique et collective* (Aubier, 1989), 223. In Taylor Adkins, "A Short List of Gilbert Simondon's Vocabulary," Fractal Ontology, 2007. https://fractalontology.wordpress.com/2007/11/28/a-short-list-of-gilbert-simondons-vocabulary/
22 Edmund Husserl, *Phenomenology and the Crisis of Philosophy*, trans. Quentin Lauer (Harper & Row, 1936/1965), 191.
23 *Le Débat*, no. 4 (September 1980), 16, 18 (trans. mine).
24 Evelyne Grossman, *The Anguish of Thought*, trans. Matthew Crispey and Louise Burchill (U. of Minnesota Press, 2018), 2, 4.
25 Josephine Wright, "Imagining a Future at a Time of Existential Threat." Presentation at New York Psychoanalytic Society and Institute, November 11, 2025.
26 Dermot Moran, *Edmund Husserl: The Crisis of the European Sciences and Transcendental Phenomenology* (Cambridge University Press, 2011), 189.
27 Moran, *Edmund Husserl: The Crisis of the European Sciences and Transcendental Phenomenology*, 7.
28 Moran, *Edmund Husserl: The Crisis of the European Sciences and Transcendental Phenomenology*, 190.
29 Sigmund Freud, "Introductory Lectures on Psycho-Analysis," *Standard Edition*, vol. 16, 371.
30 Sigmund Freud, "Totem and Taboo," *Standard Edition*, vol. 13, 158.
31 See Maureen Dowd, "Don't Kill 'Frankenstein' with Real Frankensteins at Large," *The New York Times* (May 27, 2023).
32 See Dowd, "Don't Kill 'Frankenstein' with Real Frankensteins at Large," 192.
33 See Jason Farago, "The Role of Art in a Time of War," *The New York Times* (July 28, 2022).
34 See Margo Jefferson, "On Writers and Writing; The Critic in Time of War," *The New York Times*, October 28, 2001.
35 Gaston Bachelard, *La poétique de l'espace* (Les Presses universitaires de France, 1958), 8.
36 See Alan Jasanoff, "Sick in the Head: Eric Kandel Looks at Why Certain Brains Are Hard-Wired for Mental Illness," *The New York Times Book Review* (September 23, 2018), 21.
37 François Ansermet, "The Neurobiology of Freedom." Presentation made at ThinkSwiss: Genève Meets New York, March 2, 2012.

Bibliography

Abrams, Samuel. "Disposition and the Environment." *The Psychoanalytic Study of the Child* 41, no. 1 (1986): 41–60.

Aho, Kevin. "The Uncanny in the Time of Pandemics: Heideggerian Reflections on the Coronavirus," *Existential Analysis* 32, no. 1 (2021): 5–20.

Albright, Daniel. "Series Editor's Foreword." In *Samuel Beckett and the Arts*, edited by Lois Oppenheim. London and New York: Routledge, 1999/2021.

Ansermet, François and Magistretti, Pierre. *Biology of Freedom: Neural Plasticity, Experience, and the Unconscious.* Translated by Susan Fairfield. New York: Other Press, 2007.

Auden, W.H. *Van Gogh: A Self-Portrait; Letters Revealing His Life as a Painter.* Greenwich, CT: New York Graphic Society, 1961.

Bachelard, Gaston, *The Poetics of Space* (1958), Foreword to the 1994 edition. Translated by Maria Jolas. Boston: Beacon Press, 1994.

Bachelard, Gaston. *La poétique de l'espace.* Paris: Les Presses universitaires de France, 1958.

Barrett, Lisa Feldman. "Knowledge vs. Creativity." https://iai.tv/video/knowledge-v-creativity?utm_source=YouTube&utm_medium=description

Baskin, Jason M. *Modernism beyond the Avant-Garde: Embodying Experience.* Cambridge: Cambridge University Press, 2019.

Beckett, Samuel. *The Unnamable.* New York: Grove Press, 1958.

Beckett, Samuel. *The Collected Shorter Plays of Samuel Beckett.* New York: Grove Press, 1984.

Beckett, Samuel. "Dante . . . Bruno . Vico . . Joyce." In *Disjecta*, edited by Ruby Cohn. New York: Grove Press, 1984.

Beckett, Samuel. "Henri Hayden." In *Disjecta*, edited by Ruby Cohn. New York: Grove Press, 1984.

Beckett, Samuel. "Homage to Jack B. Yeats." In *Disjecta*, edited by Ruby Cohn. New York: Grove Press, 1984.

Beckett, Samuel. "Intercessions by Denis Devlin." In *Disjecta*, edited by Ruby Cohn. New York: Grove Press, 1984.

Beckett, Samuel. "Peintres de l'Empêchement." In *Disjecta*, edited by Ruby Cohn. New York: Grove Press, 1984.

Beckett, Samuel. "La peinture des van Velde ou le monde et le pantalon." In *Disjecta*, edited by Ruby Cohn. New York: Grove Press, 1984.

Beckett, Samuel. *Company* in *NOHOW ON*. Paris, London, New York: Calder Publications. 1980/1992.

Beckett, Samuel. *Worstward Ho* in *NOHOW ON*, Paris, London, New York: Calder Publications, 1983/1992.

Beckett, Samuel. "*What is the Word*." London: Faber & Faber Ltd., 1989/2012.

Begam, Richard. *Samuel Beckett and the End of Modernity*. Stanford: Stanford University Press, 1996.

Bion, Wilfred. "Notes on Memory and Desire," *Psychoanalytic Forum* 2, no. 3 (1967): 272–273, 279–280.

Blanchot, Maurice. *The Writing of the Disaster*, translated by Ann Smock. Lincoln, NE: University of Nebraska Press, 1986/1995.

Brater, Enoch. *The Drama in the Text: Beckett's Late Fiction*. New York and Oxford: Oxford University Press, 1994.

Carhart-Harris, Robin and Friston, Karl. "The Default-Mode, Ego-Functions and Free-Energy: A Neurobiological Account of Freudian Ideas." *Brain* (February 28, 2010): 1265–1283. doi:10.1093/brain/awq010

Cary, Joyce. *Art and Reality: Ways of Creative Process*. New York: Harper & Brothers, 1958.

Caws, Mary Ann. *Symbolism, Dada, Surrealisms*. London: Reaktion Books, 2024.

Ceccatty, René de. "Le regard, le ciel et la mer." In *Geneviève Asse*, 15–19. Paris: Galerie Antoine Laurentin, 2019.

Chalmers, David. "Facing Up to the Problem of Consciousness." *Journal of Consciousness Studies* 2, no. 3 (1995): 200–219.

Clark, Andy. *Surfing Uncertainty: Prediction, Action and the Embodied Mind*. Oxford: Oxford University Press, 2016.

Clément, Bruno. *Henri Bergson, Prix Nobel de littérature*. Paris: Verdier, 2021.

Coffey, Michael. *Beckett's Children: A Literary Memoir*. New York: Evergreen Review Books, 2024.

Cott, Jonathan. "Susan Sontag: The Rolling Stone Interview,"October 4, 1979. https://www.rollingstone.com/culture/culture-news/susan-sontag-the-rolling-stone-interview-41717/4/

Damasio, Antonio. *The Feeling of What Happens*. San Diego, New York, London: Harcourt, Inc., 1999.

Damasio, Antonio. *The Strange Order of Things: Life, Feeling, and the Making of Cultures*. New York: Vintage Books, 2018.

Datta, Asijit and Boulter, Jonathan. "*Samuel Beckett and Posthuman Spaces, Textual Practice*." Jan. 16, 2025. doi:10.1080/0950236X.2025.2453645

Day, John. *John Day*. New York: Tenth Avenue Editions, Inc., 1984.

Delacampagne, Christian. "Ce qu'Occident veut dire." *Le Débat*, no. 4 (September 1980).

Dewey, John. *Democracy and Education*. New York: The Free Press, 1916.

Dowd, Maureen. "Don't Kill 'Frankenstein' with Real Frankensteins at Large." *The New York Times*, May 27, 2023.

Eagleton, Terry. "Foreword: Nothing." In *New, Beckett and Nothing: Trying to Understand Beckett*, edited by Daniela Caselli. Manchester and New York: Manchester University Press, 2010.

Esslin, Martin. *The Theatre of the Absurd*. New York: Anchor Books, 1961.

Farago, Jason. "The Role of Art in a Time of War." *The New York Times*, July 28, 2022.

Freedberg, David and Gallese, Vittorio. "Motion, Emotion and Empathy in Esthetic Experience." *TRENDS in Cognitive Sciences* 11, no. 5 (2007). doi:10.1016/j.tics.2007.02.0

Freud, Sigmund. "Three Essays on the Theory of Sexuality." In *The Standard Edition of the Complete Psychological Works of Sigmund Freud*, edited and translated by James Strachey, vol. 7 (1905), 122–245. London: Hogarth Press, 1955.

Freud, Sigmund. "Creative Writers and Day Dreaming." In *The Standard Edition of the Complete Psychological Works of Sigmund Freud*, edited and translated by James Strachey, vol. 9 (1908) [1907], 141–153. London: Hogarth Press, 1955.

Freud, Sigmund. "Leonardo Da Vinci and a Memory of His Childhood." In *The Standard Edition of the Complete Psychological Works of Sigmund Freud*, edited and translated by James Strachey, vol. 11 (1910), 57–137. London: Hogarth Press, 1955.

Freud, Sigmund. "A Note on the Unconscious in Psycho-Analysis." In *The Standard Edition of the Complete Psychological Works of Sigmund Freud*, edited and translated by James Strachey, vol. 12 (1912), 255–266. London: Hogarth Press, 1955.

Freud, Sigmund. "The Unconscious" (Appendix C, Words and Things). In *The Standard Edition of the Complete Psychological Works of Sigmund Freud*, edited and translated by James Strachey, vol. 14 (1915), 209–215. London: Hogarth Press, 1955. London: Hogarth Press, 1955.

Freud, Sigmund. "Instincts and Their Vicissitudes." In *The Standard Edition of the Complete Psychological Works of Sigmund Freud*, edited and translated by James Strachey, vol. 14 (1915), 109–140. London: Hogarth Press, 1955.

Freud. Sigmund. "Beyond the Pleasure Principle." In *The Standard Edition of the Complete Psychological Works of Sigmund Freud*, edited and translated by James Strachey, vol. 18 (1920), 7–64. London: Hogarth Press, 1955.

Freud, Sigmund. "The Ego and the Id." In *The Standard Edition of the Complete Psychological Works of Sigmund Freud*, edited and translated by James Strachey, vol. 19 (1923), 12–66. London: Hogarth Press, 1955.

Freud, Sigmund. "Dostoevsky and Parricide." In *The Standard Edition of the Complete Psychological Works of Sigmund Freud*, edited and translated by James Strachey, vol. 21 (1928) [1927], 173–196. London: Hogarth Press, 1955.

Freud, Sigmund. "Civilization and Its Discontents." In *The Standard Edition of the Complete Psychological Works of Sigmund Freud*, edited and translated by James Strachey, vol. 21 (1930) [1929], 57–145. London: Hogarth Press, 1955.

Freud, Sigmund. "The Dissection of the Psychical Personality." New Introductory Lectures on Psycho-Analysis, Lecture 31. In *The Standard Edition of the Complete Psychological Works of Sigmund Freud*, edited and translated by James Strachey, vol. 22 (1932), 57–80. London: Hogarth Press, 1955.

Freud, Sigmund. "Aphasie." In *A Moment of Transition: Two Neuroscientific Articles by Sigmund Freud*, translated and edited by Mark Solms and Michael Saling. London: The Institute of Psycho-Analysis; London and New York: Karnac Books, 1990.

Friston, Karl. "Is the Free-Energy Principle Neurocentric?," *Nature Reviews Neuroscience* 11 (2010). doi:10.1038/nrn2787-c2

Friston, Karl. "The Free-Energy Principle: A Unified Brain Theory?," *Nature Reviews Neuroscience* 11 (2010). doi:10.1038/nrn2787

Friston, Karl. "Computational Psychiatry: From Synapses to Sentience." *Molecular Psychiatry* 28 (2023): 256–268. doi:10.1038/s41380-022-01743-z

Friston, Karl and Herreros, Iñigo. "Active Inference and Learning in the Cerebellum." *Neural Computation* 28, no. 9 (2016): 1812–1839. doi:10.1162/NECO_a_00863

Gallagher, Shaun. "Empathy, Simulation, and Narrative." *Science in Context* 25, no. 3 (2012): 355–381.

Gallagher, Shaun. "Precis: Enactivist Interventions." *Philosophical Studies* 176 (2019): 803–806. doi:10.1007/s11098-018-01230-8

Gallese, Vittorio. "Visions of the Body: Embodied Simulation and Aesthetic Experience." *Aisthesis. Pratiche, linguaggi e saperi dell'estetico* 10, no. 1 (2017): 41–50. doi:10.13128/Aisthesis-20902

Gallese, Vittorio. "The Embodiment of Images: A View from the Brain-Body." Presented at Psychoanalytic Dialogues Conference, Rome, January 25, 2025.

Gallese, Vittorio. "Aesthetics and the Unconscious: Toward an Embodied Neuroscience of the Image," *JAPA*, December 4, 2025. doi:10.1177/00030651251394305

Gamwell, Lynn and Solms, Mark. *From Neurology to Psychoanalysis: Sigmund Freud's Neurological Drawings and Diagrams of the Mind*. Binghamton, NY: Binghamton University Art Museum, State University of New York, 2006.

Garelli, Jacques. *La gravitation poétique*. Paris: Mercure de France, 1966.

Garelli, Jacques. "Il y a le monde." *Esprit*, 1982.

Garelli, Jacques. *Rythmes et mondes: au revers de l'identité et de l'altérité*. Grenoble: Jérôme Million, 1991.

Garelli, Jacques. "Voir ceci et voir selon." In *Merleau-Ponty, Phénoménologie et expériences*, edited by Marc Richir and Étienne Tassin. Grenoble: Jérôme Million, 1992.

Garelli, Jacques. "Foreword: Introduction to the Problematic of Gilbert Simondon." In Gilbert Simondon, *Individuation in Light of Notions of Form and Information*, translated by Taylor Adkins. Minneapolis and London: University of Minnesota Press, 2020.

Gay, Volney Patrick. *Freud on Sublimation*. Albany, NY: State University of New York Press, 1992.

Glimcher, Arne. *Agnes Martin: Paintings, Writings, Remembrances*. New York: Phaidon, 2012.

Gori, Roland. "Science and Psychoanalysis."https://www.encyclopedia.com/psychology/dictionaries-thesauruses-pictures-and-press-releases/science-and-psychoanalysis

Goudouna, Sozita. *Beckett's Breath: Anti-Theatricality and the Visual Arts*. Edinburgh: Edinburgh University Press, 2018.

Greenberg, Clement. "The 'Crisis' of Abstract Art." In *New York: The Art World*, edited by James R. Mellow. New York: The Art Digest, 1964.

Greenberg, Clement. "The Crisis of the Easel Picture." In *Clement Greenberg, Art and Culture*. London: Beacon Press, 1961 (original version first published in *Partisan Review*, April 1948).

Grossman, Evelyne. *The Anguish of Thought*, translated by Matthew Crispey and Louise Burchill. Minneapolis: University of Minnesota Press, 2008/2018.

Grossman, Evelyne. *La créativité de la crise*. Paris: Les Éditions de Minuit, 2020.

Hellstein, Valerie. "De Kooning's Embodied Vision and Abstract Expressionism in the 1960s." In **Women Singing II* 1966 by Willem de Kooning*. London: Tate Research Publication, 2017. https://www.tate.org.uk/research/in-focus/women-singing-ii/de-koonings-embodied-vision

Hoffman, Leon. "Picasso and the Painter Model Theme: Multiple Identifications and Creative Transformations of Aggressive Conflicts." *International Review of Psycho-Analysis* 11 (1984): 291–300.

Hoffman, Leon and Oppenheim, Lois. "Three Identical Strangers and The Twinning Reaction: Clarifying History and Lessons for Today from Peter Neubauer's Twins Study." *JAMA* 322, no. 1 (2019): 10–12.

Husserl, Edmund. *Phenomenology and the Crisis of Philosophy*, translated by Quentin Lauer. New York: Harper & Row, 1936/1965.

Ishizu, Tomohiro and Zeki, Semir. "*Toward A Brain-Based Theory of Beauty*." *PLOS ONE* 6, no. 7 (2011): e21852. doi:10.1371/journal.pone.0021852

Jardine, Alice. *At the Risk of Thinking*. New York: Bloomsbury, 2020.

Jasanoff, Alan. "Sick in the Head: Eric Kandel Looks at Why Certain Brains Are Hard-Wired for Mental Illness." *The New York Times Book Review*, September 23, 2018.

Jefferson, Margo. "On Writers and Writing: The Critic in Time of War." *The New York Times*, October 28, 2001.

Johnson, Galen A."Ontology and Painting: 'Eye and Mind.'" In *The Merleau-Ponty Aesthetics Reader: Philosophy and Painting*, edited by Galen A. Johnson. Evanston, IL: Northwestern University Press, 1993.

Joyce, James. *Ulysses*. Paris: Sylvia Beach, 1922.

Judd, Donald. "New York: The Art World." In *Arts Yearbook* 7. New York: The Art Digest Inc., 1964.

Kandel, Eric. *Reductionism in Art and Brain Science*. New York: Columbia University Press, 2016.

Kesner, Ladislav. "The Predictive Mind and the Experience of the Visual Art Work." *Frontiers in Psychology* 5 (2014). doi:10.3389/fpsyg.2014.01417

Kesner, Ladislav. "A Hole in a Piece of Cardboard and Predictive Brain: The Incomprehension of Modern Art in the Light of the Predictive Coding Paradigm." *Philosophical Transactions of the Royal Society*, 2024. B 379: 20220417. doi:10.1098/rstb.2022.0417

Kramer, Hilton. "Notes on Painting in New York." In *Arts Yearbook* 7. New York: The Art Digest Inc., 1964.

Krauss, Rosalind. "Grids." *October* 9 (Summer 1979): 50–64.

Kusama, Yayoi. *Infinity Net: The Autobiography of Yayoi Kusama*. Video with interview, camera, and editing by Mary Lance. Shown in conjunction with the Agnes Martin retrospective exhibit at the Guggenheim Museum, New York. October 7, 2016–January 11, 2017.

Kuzma, Joseph. *Internet Encyclopedia of Philosophy*. https://iep.utm.edu/maurice-blanchot/#SH3b

Lange, F.P., Heilbron, M., and Kok, P. "How Do Expectations Shape Perception?," *Trends in Cognitive Sciences* 22, no. 9 (2018): 764–779.

Latour, Bruno. *Facing Gaia: Eight Lectures on the New Climatic Regime*, translated by Catherine Porter. Cambridge, UK, and Medford, MA: Polity Press, 2007.

Livio, Mario. *Why? What Makes Us Curious?* New York: Simon & Schuster, 2017.

Locatelli, Carla. *Unwording the World*. Philadelphia: University of Pennsylvania Press, 1990.

Ma, Yo Yo. "Yo Yo Ma and the Meaning of Life." Interview by David Marchese. *The New York Magazine*, November 20, 2020.

Maldiney, Henri. *Regard Parole Espace*. Lausanne: L'Âge d'homme, 1973.

Markman, Henry. "So Much Depends Upon a Red Stripe." *Psychoanalytic Inquiry* 44, no. 4 (2024): 398–409. doi:10.1080/07351690.2024.2345588

Marom, Shimon. "Dialogue across Chasm: Are Psychology and Neurophysiology Incompatible?," *Neuron* 107 (August 19, 2020): 600–602.

Martin, Agnes. "Beauty is the Mystery of Life." 1989. https://www.artbook.com/blog-excerpt-agnes-martin-beauty-is-the-mystery-of-life.html

Merleau-Ponty, Maurice. *Le Visible et l'Invisible*. Paris: Gallimard, 1964.

Merleau-Ponty, Maurice. "Indirect Language and the Voices of Silence." In *The Prose of the World*, Edited by Claude Lefort, translated by John O'Neill. Evanston, IL: Northwestern University Press, 1973.

Merleau-Ponty, Maurice. "Cézanne's Doubt." In *The Merleau-Ponty Aesthetics Reader: Philosophy and Painting*, edited by Galen A. Johnson. Evanston, IL: Northwestern University Press, 1945/1993.

Merleau-Ponty, Maurice. "Eye and Mind." In *The Merleau-Ponty Aesthetics Reader: Philosophy and Painting*, edited by Galen A. Johnson. Evanston, IL: Northwestern University Press, 1961/1993.

Merleau-Ponty, Maurice. "Eye and Mind." In *The Primacy of Perception*, edited by James M. Edie (Evanston, IL: Northwestern University Press, 1964).

Moorjani, Angela. "Genesis, Child's Play, and the Gaze of Silence: Samuel Beckett and Paul Klee." *Samuel Beckett Today/Aujourd'hui* 19 (2008): 187–297.

Moran, Dermot. *Edmund Husserl: The Crisis of the European Sciences and Transcendental Phenomenology: An Introduction*. Cambridge: Cambridge University Press, 2011.

Muth, Claudia and Carbon, Claus-Christian. "Ambivalence of Artistic Photographs Stimulates Interest and the Motivation to Engage." *Psychology of Aesthetics, Creativity, and the Arts* 18, no. 3 (2024): 287–302. doi:10.1037/aca0000448

Muth, Claudia, Hesslinger, Vera M., and Carbon, Claus-Christian. "The Appeal of Challenge in the Perception of Art: How Ambiguity, Solvability of Ambiguity, and the Opportunity for Insight Affect Appreciation." *Psychology of Aesthetics, Creativity, and the Arts* 9, no. 3 (2015): 206–216. doi:10.1037/a0038814

Muth, Claudia, Raab, Marius Hans, and Carbon, Claus-Christian. "Expecting the Unexpected: How Gallery Visitors Experience Semantic Instability in Art." *Art & Perception* 5 (2017): 121–142. doi:10.1163/22134913-00002062

Muth, Claudia, Westphal-Fitch, Gesche and Carbon, Claus-Christian. "Seeking (Dis)order: Ordering Appeals but Slight Disorder and Complex Order Trigger Interest." *Psychology of Aesthetics, Creativity, and the Arts* 15, no. 3 (2021): 439–457. doi:10.1037/aca0000284

Nagel, Thomas. "What Is It Like To Be a Bat?," *The Philosophical Review* 83, no. 4 (1974): 435–450.

Noudelmann, François. "What Do Jean-Paul and Simone de Beauvoir Have to Say to Us Today?," *Diogenes* 54, no. 216 (2007): 35–39.

Noy, Pinchas and Noy-Sharav, Dorit. "Art and Emotions." *International Journal of Applied Psychoanalytic Studies* 10, no. 2 (2013): 100–107.

Ogden, Thomas. *The Primitive Edge of Experience*. Northvale, NJ, and London: Jason Aronson, 1989.

Ogden, Thomas. "Ontological Psychoanalysis or 'What Do You Want To Be When You Grow Up?,'" *The Psychoanalytic Quarterly* 88, no. 4 (2019): 661–684. doi:10.1080/00332828.2019.1656928

Ogden, Thomas H. "Rethinking the Concepts of the Unconscious and Analytic Time." *JAPA* 69, no. 1 (2021): 1–17.

Oppenheim, Lois. *The Painted Word: Samuel Beckett's Dialogue with Art.* Ann Arbor: The University of Michigan Press, 2000.

Oppenheim, Lois. *A Curious Intimacy: Art and Neuro-Psychoanalysis.* London and New York: Routledge, 2005.

Oppenheim, Lois. "The Lexicographer's Nightmare." In *From the Couch to the Lab: Trends in Psychodynamic Neuroscience*, edited by Aikaterini Fotopoulou, Donald Pfaff, and Martin Conway, 282–292. Oxford: Oxford University Press, 2012.

Oppenheim, Lois. "Review of Neubauer Twin Study: An Interview about a Controversy or a Controversial Interview?," *International Journal of Controversial Discussions* 1 (2020): 171–188.

Oppenheim, Lois. "Commentary on Mark Solms' 'New Project for a Scientific Psychology,'" *Neuropsychoanalysis* 22, no. 1–2 (2021): 87–89. doi:10.1080/15294145.2021.1878617

Panksepp, Jaak. *Affective Neuroscience: The Foundations of Human and Animal Emotions.* New York and Oxford: Oxford University Press, 1998.

Panksepp, Jaak. "Emotional Foundations of Creativity: The Brain's SEEKING System." In *Secrets of Creativity: What Neuroscience, the Arts, and Our Minds Reveal*, edited by Suzanne Nalbantian and Paul M. Matthews. Oxford: Oxford Academic, 2019.

Panksepp, Jaak and Biven, Lucy. *The Archeology of Mind: Neuroevolutionary Origins of Human Emotions.* New York and London: W.W. Norton, 2012.

Panksepp, Jaak and Trevarthen, Colwyn. "The Neuroscience of Emotion in Music." In *Communicative Musicality: Exploring the Basis of Human Companionship*, 105–146. Oxford: Oxford University Press, 2009.

Pepperell, Robert. "Being Alive to the World: An Artist's Perspective on Predictive Processing." *Philosophical Transactions of the Royal Society*, 2023. doi:10.1098/rstb.2022.0429

Perloff, Marjorie. "Modernism after Postmodernism." Presentation at The Center for the Creative and the Critical, Ashoka University and literaryactivism.com, in partnership with The Oxford Research Centre (TORCH) and the India International Centre, Delhi, 2022.

Princenthal, Nancy, "With Her Back to the World and Her Face to the Camera." *Brooklyn Rail*, November 2013. https://brooklynrail.org/2013/11/criticspage/with-her-back-to-the-world-and-her-face-to-the-camera/

Princenthal, Nancy. *Agnes Martin: Her Life and Art.* New York and London: Thames & Hudson, 2015.

Putman, Jacques and Juliet, Charles. *Bram van Velde.* Paris: Maeght, 1975.

Raviv, Shaun, "The Genius Neuroscientist Who Might Hold the Key to True AI."https://www.wired.com/story/karl-friston-free-energy-principle-artificial-intelligence/

Ricoeur, Paul. *Freud & Philosophy: An Essay on Interpretation*, translated by Denis Savage. New Haven: Yale University Press, 1970.

Rodman, Selden. *Conversations with Artists.* New York: Delvin-Adair Co., 1957.

Rose, Gilbert J. *Necessary Illusion: Art as Witness.* Madison, CT: International Universities Press, Inc., 1996.

Rose, Gilbert J. *Between Couch and Piano: Psychoanalysis, Music, Art and Neuroscience.* Hove and New York: Brunner Routledge, 2004.

Rothko, Christopher. "Introduction." In Mark Rothko, *The Artist's Reality*, xi–xxxi. New Haven and London: Yale University Press, 2004.

Rothko, Christopher. *Mark Rothko: From the Inside Out*. New Haven and London: Yale University Press, 2015. doi:10.12987/9780300212815-004

Salisbury, Laura. "'What Is the Word': Beckett's Aphasic Modernism," *Journal of Beckett Studies* 17, no. 1–2 (2009): 78–126. doi:10.3366/E0309520709000090

Sartre, Jean-Paul. *L'Existentialisme est un humanisme*. Paris: Les Éditions Nagel, 1946.

Sartre, Jean-Paul. *Qu'est-ce que la littérature?* Paris: Gallimard, 1948.

Sartre, Jean-Paul. *What is Literature?* Translated by Bernard Frechtman. New York: Philosophical Library, 1949.

Sbriscia-Fioretti, Beatrice, Berchio, Cristina, Freedberg, David, Gallese, Vittorio, and Umiltà, Maria Alessandra. "ERP Modulation during Observation of Abstract Paintings by Franz Kline." *PLoS ONE* 8 (2013). doi:10.1371/journal.pone.0075241

Schiller, Britt-Marie. "Figurability in the Art of Louise Bourgeois." *American Imago* 81, no. 3 (2024): 305–333.

Schjeldahl, Peter. "Drawing Lines." *The New Yorker*, October 17, 2016.

Seth, Anil K. "Interoceptive Inference, Emotion, and the Embodied Self." *Trends in Cognitive Sciences* 17, no. 11 (2013): 565–573.

Seth, Anil K. and Friston, Karl J."Active Interoceptive Inference and the Emotional Brain." *Philosophical Transactions of the Royal Society*, 2016. B37120160007. doi:10.1098/rstb.2016.0007

Simondon, Gilbert. *L'Individu et sa genèse physico-biologique*. Paris: Presses Universitaires de France, 1964/1995.

Simondon, Gilbert. *Individuation in Light of Notions of Form and Information*, translated by Taylor Adkins. Minneapolis: University of Minnesota Press, 2005/2020.

Skelton, Ross M. *The Edinburgh International Encyclopaedia of Psychoanalysis*. Edinburgh: Edinburgh University Press, 2006.

Solms, Mark. "The Conscious Id." *Neuropsychoanalysis* 15, no. 1 (2013): 5–19.

Solms, Mark. "Consciousness by Surprise," *Journal of Integrative Neuroscience* 13 (2014): 173–185.

Solms, Mark. "A Neuropsychoanalytic Approach to the Hard Problem of Consciousness." *Journal of Integrative Neuroscience* 13, no. 2 (2014): 173–185. doi:10.1142/S0219635214400032

Solms, Mark. "Empathy as Developmental Achievement: Beyond Embodied Simulation." In *Neuroscience and Critique*, edited by and Ed Pluth. London and New York: Routledge, 2016.

Solms, Mark. "Consciousness by Surprise: A Neuropsychoanalytic Approach to the Hard Problem." In *Biophysics of Consciousness: A Foundational Approach*, edited by Roman Poznanski, Jack Tuszynski, and Todd E. Feinberg, 129–148. New York: World Scientific, 2016.

Solms, Mark. "The Neurobiological Underpinnings of Psychoanalytic Theory and Therapy." *Frontiers in Behavioral Neuroscience* 12, article 294 (2018). doi:10.3389/fnbeh.2018.00294

Solms, Mark. "The Hard Problem of Consciousness and the Free Energy Principle." *Frontiers in Psychology* 9, article 2714 (January 2019): 7.

Solms, Mark. "New Project for a Scientific Psychology: General Scheme." *Neuropsychoanalysis* 22, no. 1–2 (2020): 5–35. doi:10.1080/15294145.2020.1833361

Solms, Mark. *The Hidden Spring: A Journey to the Source of Consciousness*. London and New York: W.W. Norton, 2021.

Solms, Mark. "Revision of Drive Theory," *JAPA* 69, no. 6 (2021): 1033–1091.

Solms, Mark. "'Function' in Functional Neurological Disorders: The Common Ground of Neuroscience and Psychoanalysis." *Neuropsychoanalysis* 27, no. 1 (2025): 5–18. doi:10.1080/15294145.2025.2472340

Solms, Mark. *The Only Cure: Freud and the Neuroscience of Mental Healing*. London: Weidenfeld & Nicholson, 2026.

Solms, Mark and Friston, Karl. "How and Why Consciousness Arises," *Journal of Consciousness Studies* 25, no. 5–6(2018), 202–238.

Solms, Mark and Turnbull, Oliver. *The Brain and the Inner World*. New York: Other Press, 2010.

Solms, Mark and Turnbull, Oliver. "What Is Neuropsychoanalysis?," *Neuropsychoanalysis* 13, no. 2 (2011): 133–145.

Solms, Mark and Zellner, Margaret R. "Freudian Affect Theory Today." In *From the Couch to the Lab: Trends in Psychodynamic Neuroscience*, edited by Aikaterini Fotopoulou, Donald Pfaff, and Martin Conway, 5–28. Oxford: Oxford University Press, 2012.

Sontag, Susan. *Against Interpretation*. New York: Farrar, Straus and Giroux, 1961.

Soutif, Daniel. "Flight into Whiteness: Bram Van Velde." *Art Forum*, Summer 1990. https://www.artforum.com/features/flight-into-whiteness-bram-van-velde-204814/

Stevens, Victoria. "To Think without Thinking: The Implications of Combinatory Play and the Creative Process for Neuroaesthetics." *American Journal of Play* 7, no. 1 (2014): 99–119.

Sulloway, Frank J. *Freud, Biologist of the Mind*. New York: Basic Books, 1979.

Supervielle, Silvia Baron. "Le temps arrêté." In *Geneviève Asse*. Plomelin: Éditions Palantines, 2004.

Supervielle, Silvia Baron. "Approches de l'aube." In *Geneviève Asse*, 10–11. Paris: Galerie Antoine Laurentin, 2019.

Van de Cruys, Sander, Bervoets, Jo, and Moors, Agnes. "Preferences Need Inferences: Learning, Valuation, and Curiosity in Aesthetic Experience." In *The Routledge International Handbook of Neuroaesthetics*, edited by Marcos Nadal and Martin Skov, 475–506. London and New York: Routledge, 2023.

Van de Cruys, Sander, Frascaroli, Jacopo, and Friston, Karl. "Order and Change in Art: Towards an Active Inference Account of Aesthetic Experience." *Philosophical Transactions of the Royal Society*, 2023. B379:20220411. doi:10.1098/rstb.2022.0411

Van de Cruys, Sander and Wagemans, Johan. "Putting Reward in Art: A Tentative Error Account of Visual Art." *I-Perception* 2 (2011): 1035–1062.

Vessel, Edward A., Starr, Gabrielle G., and Rubin, Nava. "Art Reaches Within: Aesthetic Experience, the Self and the Default Mode Network." *Frontiers in Neuroscience*, 2013. doi:10.3389/fnins.2013.00258

Wilson, Laurie. "Alberto Giacometti's Woman with Her Throat Cut: Multiple Meanings and Methodology." *The Annual of Psychoanalysis* 26 (1999): 143–172.

Zatorre, Robert J. and Salimpoor, Valorie N."Why Music Makes Our Brain Sing." *The New York Times*, June 7, 2013.

Index